CANNABIS
TRIPS

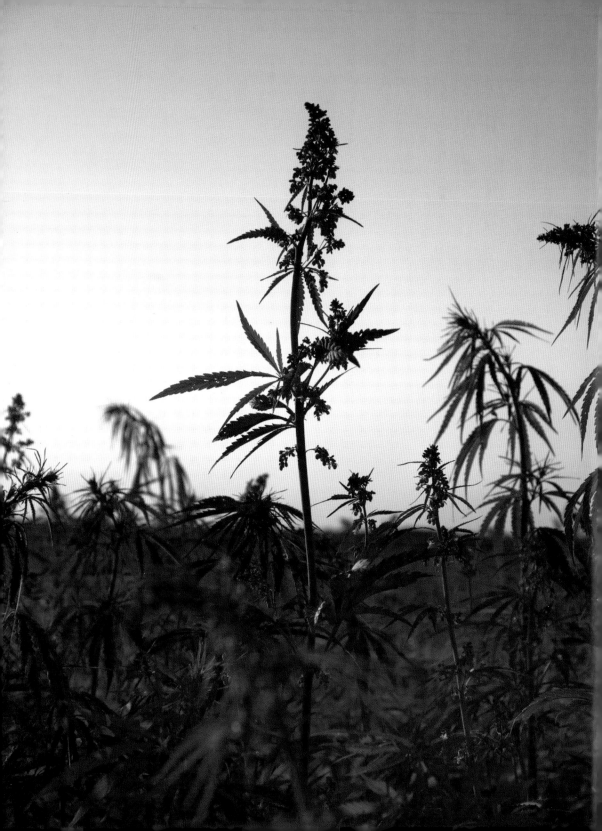

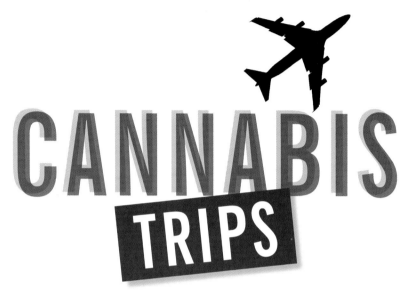

CANNABIS TRIPS

A GLOBAL GUIDE THAT LEAVES NO TURN UNSTONED

by Bill Weinberg

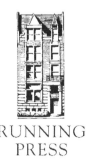

RUNNING
PRESS

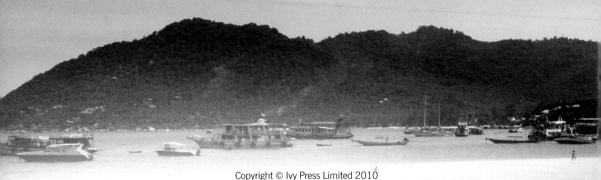

Library of Congress Control Number: 2009938622

ISBN: 978-0-7624-3812-9

This book was created by

Ivy Press
210 High Street, Lewes
East Sussex BN7 2NS, UK
www.ivy-group.co.uk

CREATIVE DIRECTOR Peter Bridgewater
PUBLISHER Jason Hook
EDITORIAL DIRECTOR Tom Kitch
ART DIRECTOR Wayne Blades
DESIGNER Clare Barber
PICTURE RESEARCHER Katie Greenwood

AUTHOR'S NOTE
'As nature has given light and day free to all, so all lands are open to the brave.'
TACITUS, THE HISTORIES, BOOK IV

Dedicated to Brian Hill, freedom fighter,
and my Emerald Triangle tour guide.

PUBLISHER'S NOTE
We take great care to ensure that the information included in this book is accurate
and presented in good faith, but no warranty is provided. This material is intended
for informational and entertainment purposes only. The publisher does not condone
illegal activity of any kind.

Running Press Book Publishers
2300 Chestnut Street, Philadelphia,
PA 19103-4371

Visit us on the web!
www.runningpress.com

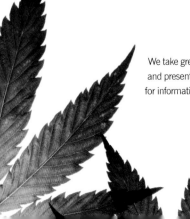

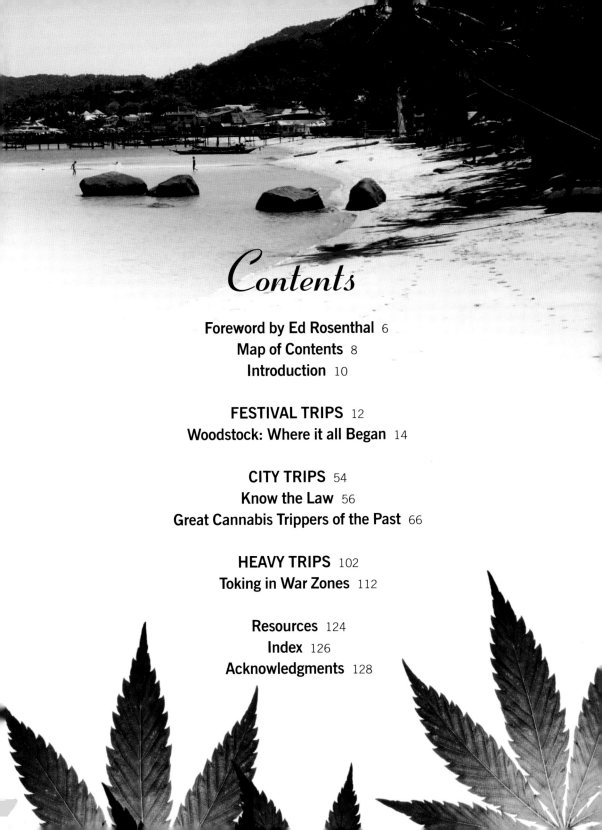

Contents

FOREWORD

Marijuana use is ubiquitous worldwide. It cuts across national boundaries and attracts people of all ages, genders, and cultural backgrounds into its swirling stream of altered consciousness. It changes the way people think rather than what they think, so it subtly modifies perceptions.

Marijuana has the remarkable ability to help you see beyond the surface into the essence and ephemeral, but it tells no lies and helps reveal reality. Rick James sang of the experience, "I'm in love with Mary Jane… And when I'm feeling low she comes as no surprise. Turns me on with her love. Takes me to paradise." Rick was talking about thinking without the blinders and filters we learn to use to view the world.

Since it has such a profound effect it is no wonder that marijuana users seek important sites, events and celebrations in a tradition as old as Chaucer, whose pilgrims "seken strange strondes [shores]… in sondry londes [lands]." Both groups journey to sacred places to celebrate their chosen paths.

It is a sign of the times that this book was written and published and will be used. It's an indication of cannabis culture's maturation and acceptance by much of mainstream society. *Cannabis Trips* is the essential guidebook for the marijuana-motivated traveler. It offers thorough descriptions of the scenes, their surroundings, their highs and lows, inside information, essential tips, and serious warnings and considerations.

It answers the questions: Why is this journey important? Why should I go? Does the climate suit my clothes? Is this trip for me?

I have attended some of the events and visited some of the cities and areas described in this book. I find the author provides an accurate and well-nuanced view of what to expect. This book will be a useful guide in my future travels.

Ed Rosenthal, November 2009

MAP OF CONTENTS

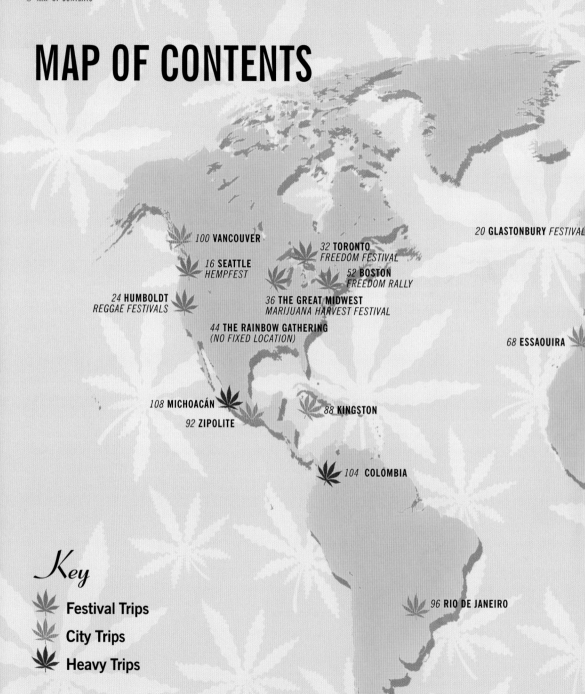

Key

Festival Trips

City Trips

Heavy Trips

INTRODUCTION

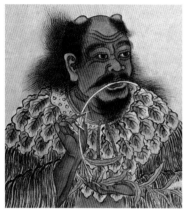

Shen Nung tested hundreds of herbs for their medical properties—luckily for him, one of them was cannabis.

5,000 YEARS OF CANNABIS TRAVELERS

As with all useful plants, the history of cannabis is inextricably linked with human travel. First growing in Central Asia—also the home of onions, garlic, and cotton—cannabis followed human migrations into China and India, where more resinous strains were developed for their medicinal application.

The first apparent written reference to cannabis was in the now-lost botanical compendium compiled by the Chinese emperor Shen Nung (c. 2800 BCE), and the earliest confirmed written reference was in the Hindu *Atharva Veda*, which noted *bhanga* as among the "kingdoms of herbs which release us from anxiety."

Nomadic peoples helped to disperse the plant from Asia into the West. The Greek historian Herodotus noted in around 450 BCE that the Scythians would throw cannabis on the red-hot stones of their sweat lodges and then be "transported by the vapor." Many believe the Bible's references to *kaneh* or *kaneh bosm* that are often translated to calamus or sweet cane actually denote cannabis.

Cannabis became widespread throughout the Islamic world. Kif-toking survived the Christian reconquest of Spain, albeit underground, and first entered the New World on Spanish galleons. In 1800, Napoleon Bonaparte issued an order to his troops in Egypt not to drink "certain Muslim beverages made with hashish" or "to inhale the smoke from seeds [sic] of hashish." That he had to issue this order is evidence that many did. After this, a vogue for hashish caught on among French poets and intellectuals—the very first seeds of what would explode as the counterculture of the 1960s. So the Californian cannabis cultivators who journeyed to Afghanistan for potent seeds in the 1970s were continuing in a tradition that goes back millennia.

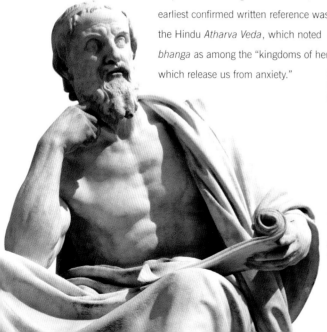

Herodotus knew about cannabis, but we don't know if he actually inhaled.

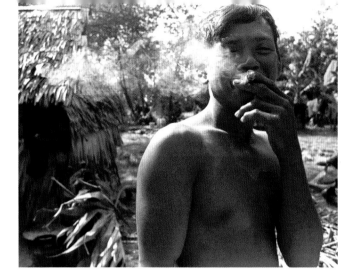

TOURISM AND THE GLOBAL CANNABIS CULTURE

Western counterculture is increasingly merging with the traditions of places with long histories of use of the plant to form a global cannabis culture. The catch-all word "drugs" conflates the natural herb cannabis with deadly, addictive, and highly processed white powders such as heroin and cocaine—and conservatives are trying to overturn Europe's decriminalization policies and disparage what they call "drug tourism". But for millions all around the world, cannabis enhances life. However, all drugs are subject to abuse, and herbally hip travelers should be good emissaries of the global cannabis culture—stoners being stupid and disrespectful is propaganda for the prohibitionist backlash. Know the law and have some savvy about the political realities of your destination.

OTHER DESTINATIONS

This book will just give you a taste of what to expect in a few cannabis havens, but there are plenty of others. In Europe, Prague and Sarajevo have burgeoning cannabis scenes, and various places in the Middle East and Asia may lure the more adventurous travelers. Lebanon is famous for its hashish, while in Pakistan, although thoroughly illegal, cannabis is widely used by pilgrims at the shrines of Sufi saints. Cannabis became freely available in Cambodia following the fall

of the Khmer Rouge in 1978, and you can still get "happy soup" in the marketplace in Phnom Penh, although the scene is nowhere near as loose as it was just a decade ago.

Hawaii, that crossroads of the Pacific, is up there with Humboldt and Amsterdam as a center of high-quality cultivation and genetic innovation. Belize, with a strong Rasta culture, has plentiful herb, and Argentina, while not a major producer, has become something of a cannabis haven since decriminalizing in 2008. There are also other festivals in America such as the July 4 Smoke-In in Washington DC and the May Day affair in New York City, now the premier event of the Global Marijuana March (a series of rallies held in different parts of the world around the first Saturday of May).

But, wherever you go, if cannabis is one of the motivations for your journeys, be a hip traveler not a clueless tourist—and be a good ambassador for the herb.

So long Khmer Rouge, hello "happy soup." Although not the haven it once was, Cambodia's Phnom Penh market is still a place where cannabis can be found.

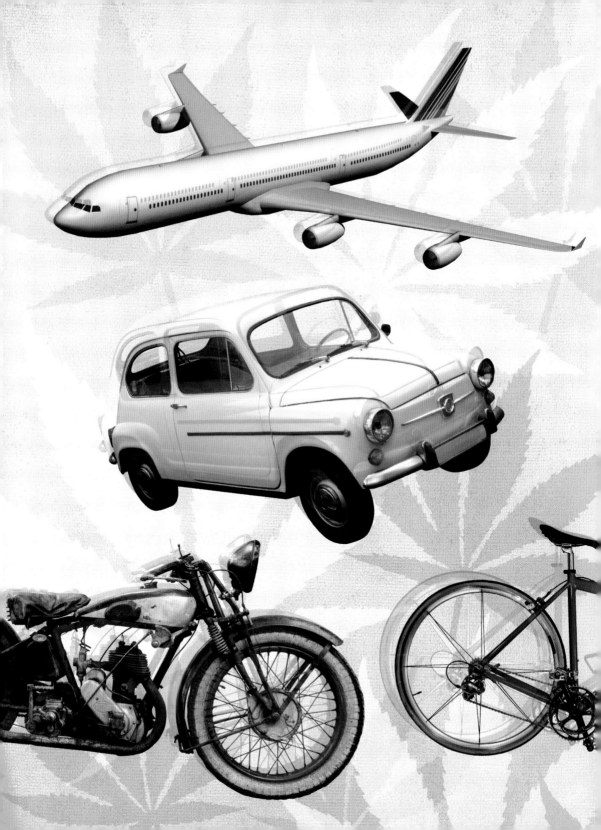

FESTIVAL TRIPS

Festivals and marijuana—they're inseparable. It might have all started with the music festivals of the late 1960s—and of course Woodstock is widely considered the grand-daddy of them all—but there is now an increasing number of festivals around the world, the sole (or soul) purpose of which is to celebrate the world of weed. Of course music festivals are still big fixtures on the counterculture calendar, but nowadays featuring fewer confused naked people. The times, they are a-changin'.

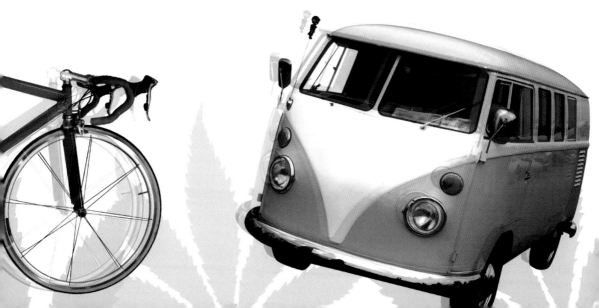

Woodstock: Where it all Began

Woodstock Music and Art Fair, August 15–18, 1969, was billed as "Three Days of Peace and Music," and it went on to become the symbol of a generation. But it took just about everyone by surprise.

The festival was named after a town in upstate New York's Catskill Mountains. The area around the town had long been popular with artists, and Bob Dylan and the Band and Jimi Hendrix were living in the region in 1969. The first site was Wallkill, Orange County, some

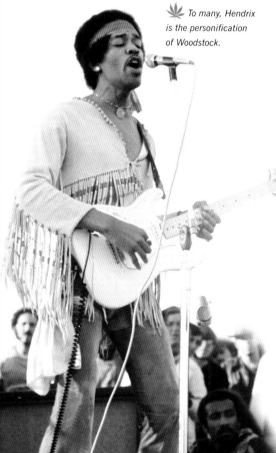

To many, Hendrix is the personification of Woodstock.

60 miles (100 kilometers) south of Woodstock. Problems with the town fathers prompted the promoters to seek another location at the last minute in Bethel, Sullivan County. The initial Bethel venue proved too small, and the conservative townsfolk were not cooperative—then dairy farmer Max Yasgur stepped forward and offered the use of his land. The show was on.

Farmer Yasgur famously told the crowd from the stage: "You've proven to the world...that a half million young people can get together and have three days of fun and music, and have nothing *but* fun and music and I God Bless You for it!" And half a million it was. Most were gatecrashers, but after a certain point nobody cared. It soon became clear that Woodstock had transcended a mere rock concert—and, needless to say, the air throughout was thick with cannabis smoke.

Local services were overwhelmed, and the gathered multitudes were left to manage the virtual city that had grown up in the rain and mud of the big cow pasture for themselves. The hippie humanitarian Wavy Gravy and his Hog Farm Commune rose to the occasion, building kitchens and shelters. After the event—which featured performances by many of the premier rock and folk acts of the day, including The Who, Joan Baez, Country Joe and the Fish, John Sebastian, Ravi Shankar, the Grateful Dead, Creedence Clearwater Revival, Sly and the Family

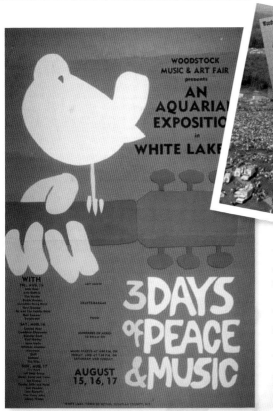

Woodstock became a city of 500,000 people for a weekend—for $18.00 each!

A white dove reinforces the message of peace on this promotional poster.

Stone, Jimi Hendrix, Janis Joplin, Santana, Canned Heat, Ten Years After, the Band (then Dylan's back-up band, although Bob himself was a no-show), Joe Cocker, the Paul Butterfield Blues Band, and Crosby, Stills, Nash, and Young—the spirit of cooperation and brotherhood continued as the 600-acre (240-hectare) cleanup was accomplished in less than five days by the Woodstock crew and concert attendees.

As a generation-defining mega-event, the spirit of Woodstock lives on. A 25th-anniversary concert in Saugerties, NY, a short distance from Woodstock,

was a success, bringing back Country Joe McDonald, John Sebastian, Santana—and Bob Dylan this time! However, a 1999 30th-anniversary concert near Rome, NY, was marred by a violent post-concert riot, attributed by some to excessive commercialism (even charging for water)—a stark contrast to the original event.

Closer to the real Woodstock spirit—although minus the drug use—is the annual Harvest Festival that the Bethel Woods Center for the Arts holds on the site of the original 1969 festival. The festival is held each Sunday from late August to the Columbus Day weekend. With arts-and-crafts workshops, wine tasting, gourmet vegetarian food, and—mostly—acoustic music, this is the manifestation of the best of the Woodstock generation, mellowed with age but true to its ideals. Admission is free.

SEATTLE
HEMPFEST **USA**

Seattle is the quintessential Pacific Rim city, magnificently situated on a narrow strip of land surrounded by towering mountains, the ocean, and Lake Washington. The "Emerald City" is one of the centers of alternative culture in America.

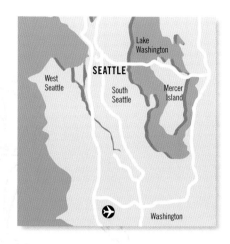

Seattle's Hempfest is the largest cannabis policy reform event in the world—the protestival's messages comfortably rubbing shoulders with a fun festival atmosphere.

The birthplace of grunge and matrix of Nirvana was also the scene of the world-shaking protests of November 1999 against the World Trade Organization. Since 1991, Seattle has hosted what has grown into the USA's biggest cannabis festival.

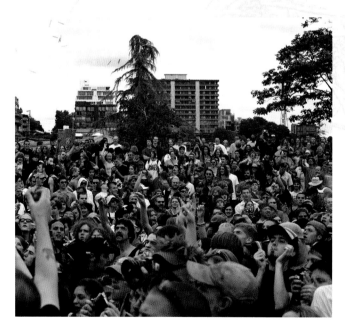

THE HIGHS

High-quality indoor hydroponic cannabis abounds, although it is not cheap, and there is no shortage of spectacular scenery. Go to the top of the 600-foot (180-meter) Space Needle built for the 1962 World's Fair and get the lay of the land. Two jewels of the USA's National Parks system are clearly visible on a sunny day: inland and to the south lies Mt. Rainier, the highest peak in the Cascades at 14,400 feet (4,390 meters)—perennially snow-crowned and dominating the landscape; across Puget Sound to the west of the Space Needle rise the Olympics, capping their green peninsula with white-tipped peaks cloaked in coniferous rainforest.

In addition to being an ideal base for mountain treks, Seattle has plenty to offer the alternative traveler. Cruise the Pike Place Market for some fresh salmon or local organic produce, then check out nearby Left Bank

Books, the local anarchist infoshop, to read up on Seattle's radical history—like the February 1919 general strike that brought the city to a complete halt for a week. Vegetarian cuisine abounds, with the most popular such eateries including Araya's Vegetarian Place in the University District and the Café Flora in the Capitol Hill neighborhood. Capitol Hill, on the city's east side, is something of an alternative enclave, with lots of funky coffee shops and the like. Across Interstate 5 to the west, the Wallingford district hosts the Terra Hemp store at 4419 Wallingford Avenue North, which boasts a wide selection of all-natural fiber goods.

Another draw is the Bumbershoot alternative music and art festival, held each September at the Seattle Center, also built for the World's Fair. The name is from the local lingo for "umbrella," an all-too-appropriate symbol for the city. Which brings us to the city's climate.

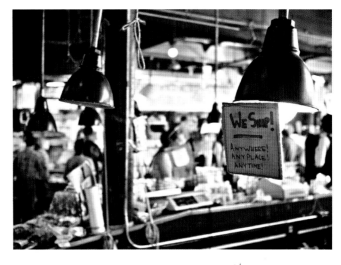

THE LOWS

Seattle has magnificent weather for a tantalizing few weeks of summer; the rest of the year the city is subject to more or less daily rain and mist. The average number of clear Seattle days per year is around fifty. Like most American cities, it has been subject to runaway gentrification over the past twenty years, meaning prices can often be high.

Munchies anyone? Pike Place Market is home to one of America's oldest farmers' markets.

Get high in Seattle—Space Needle affords breathtaking views of the spectacular scenery that surrounds the city.

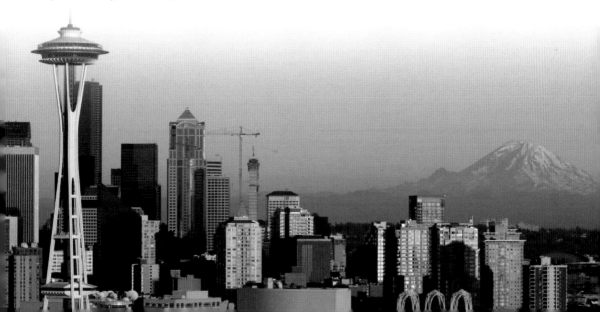

THE DOPE

The best is the famous BC Bud, the hydroponic sativa-indica hybrid that comes in from British Columbia across the border to the north; this is also the priciest. Emerald Triangle outdoor Kush varieties from Northern California are also highly rated, although they have increasingly been pushed from the market by the BC product in recent years. There is some quality indoor growing going on in Seattle and the environs as well, as the weather does not favor an outdoor crop. As throughout the West Coast, compacted Mexican is also available at a fraction of the price (and potency).

THE FESTIVAL

Originally billed in 1991 as the "Washington Hemp Expo," Seattle Hempfest has grown from a homespun affair of a few hundred participants to a counterculture extravaganza that draws over 100,000 visitors every August. It now has multiple stages spread along Elliott and Myrtle Edwards parks on the waterfront, with scores of bands performing over two days. Part cultural celebration and part political rally, it features hundreds of vendors selling legal hemp products as well as the requisite munchies, literature, hand-blown glass bongs, and the like. Past performers include hard rockers Mos Generator, British reggae artist Pato Banton, Latin hip-hop band Los Marijuanos, and Seattle's political songster Jim Page, who has long been a fixture. Speakers have included Seattle City Council member Nick Licata, former Seattle Police Chief Norm Stamper, actor Woody Harrelson, author and activist Ed Rosenthal, medical-marijuana pioneer Dennis Peron, and crusading industrial-hemp advocate Jack Herer.

One of the many stages at Hempfest 2006, where speakers, such as actor-activist Woody Harrelson, and songsters unite under the decriminalization message.

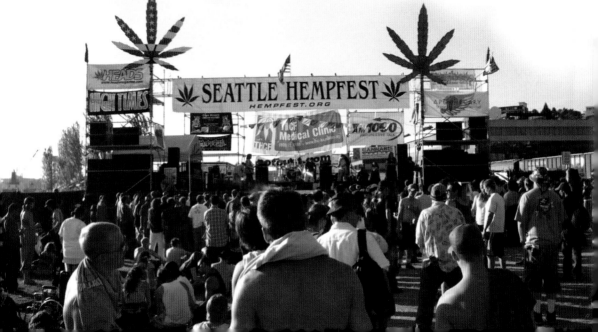

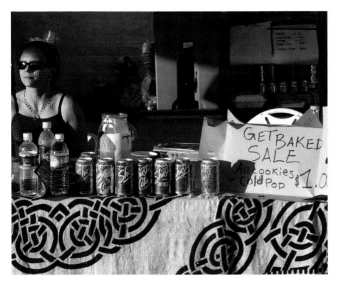

KNOW THE LAW

Depending on the amounts involved, possession of cannabis in Washington State is punishable by a possible jail term and/or a fine. Cultivation and sale is even more likely to incur a heavy penalty. However, Seattle voters in 2003 passed an initiative making adult marijuana possession offenses the lowest law-enforcement priority, which makes for a relatively tolerant atmosphere in the city.

Washington voters approved a ballot initiative legalizing use of medical marijuana in 1998. This requires a doctor's recommendation and a legitimate medical use, for example to relieve the symptoms of glaucoma.

In 1994, the organizers had to enter into negotiations brokered by the local chapter of the American Civil Liberties Union before the city would give the fast-growing event a permit. In 2006 the city fathers again balked, and the organizers—led by the festival's director Vivian McPeak—ended up going to court. But accommodations were arrived at, and Hempfest is still going strong.

Stall vendors abound, selling everything from pot paraphernalia to cookies.

There have been a few busts at Hempfest in recent years, and attendees are strongly urged not to buy (or sell) cannabis at the festival. A lot of smoking goes on, especially along the waterfront, although the cops are mostly looking for drug dealers rather than smokers. Still, those who wish to smoke should be reasonably discreet—Washington is not one of the few states that have decriminalized marijuana.

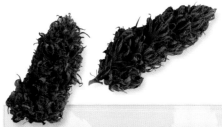

Dope Sheet

THE PRODUCT: If money's no object, the hydroponically grown BC Bud is the smoke of choice; outdoor varieties from Northern California also make an appearance.

LOOK OUT FOR: Vegetarian cuisine; farmers' markets; take time out of the city and go on any of the numerous mountain treks for scenery that will take your breath away.

GLASTONBURY FESTIVAL UK

The organizers of the Glastonbury Festival actively discourage the dealing and use of drugs at the event. But historically the festival, held in June on the meadows of Worthy Farm, Somerset, has been an essential part of the UK's alternative calendar.

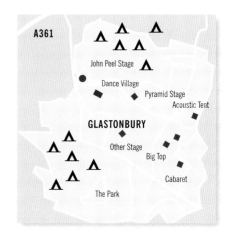

The first big rock festival on the farm, which is situated in the mythical Vale of Avalon, was the Glastonbury Fayre of 1971. David Bowie headlined, and it drew 12,000. It was revived in 1978 as the Festival of Contemporary Performing Arts and quickly grew after that, today drawing 170,000.

THE HIGHS

Glastonbury town – situated 11 kilometres (7 miles) from the festival site – and the surrounding area are steeped in the deep history of Britain, and the alternative culture that today surrounds the locale has a tinge of neopaganism and nostalgia for the pre-Christian world.

Glastonbury Tor, a hill overlooking the town, is held by local lore to have been the home of Gwyn ap Nudd, Fairy King and Lord of the Underworld. St Michael's Tower, which tops the Tor, is the surviving remnant of a medieval church and monastery, an adjunct to the now ruined abbey in the town.

Because it had been a sacred site since Neolithic times, Glastonbury became an early centre of Christianity in Britain, and to keep the pilgrims coming, the monks there invented a lively local history. Joseph of Arimathea is said to have arrived after the Crucifixion bearing the Holy Grail, which he kept in an oratory he built on

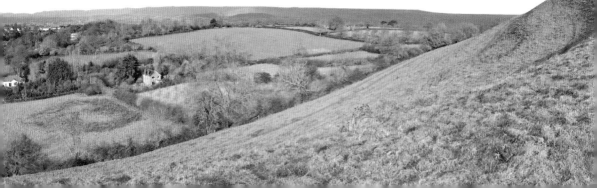

the Tor—and St Patrick was said to have established a hermitage on its ruins after his return from Ireland. On Wirral Hill, Joseph of Arimathea is also supposed to have driven his staff into the ground, which miraculously took root and blossomed into the Glastonbury Thorn, a hawthorn tree revered by pilgrims for centuries. The tree died in 1991, although some say the original tree had been destroyed during the English Civil War.

Glastonbury and the Vale of Avalon have long been associated with the legendary King Arthur. Some 19 miles (30 kilometers) south of Glastonbury lies Cadbury Castle, a place with the best claim to being the Camelot of Arthurian romance. Locals claim to see the ghosts of Arthur and his knights riding above the hill on Midsummer's Eve.

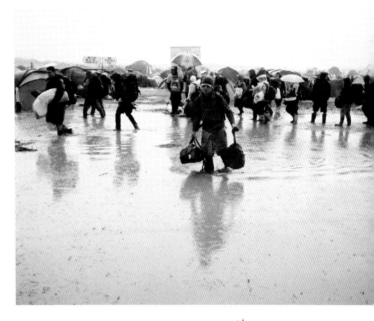

All of this fit with the prevailing alternative ethos of the late 1960s and early 1970s and made the area an obvious choice for a festival that celebrated the counterculture. The massive, commercial event that we have today still has some of that ethos driving it.

THE LOWS
The weather can be rainy, and more than once the grounds have been turned into quagmires. And as this is dairy country, there's no shortage of cow droppings…

Early summer in England's West Country can be notoriously wet. "If it's raining it must be Glastonbury weekend," goes the saying.

Glastonbury Tor is steeped in history and legend—and a visit to this famous Somerset landmark only helps to reinforce its mystique.

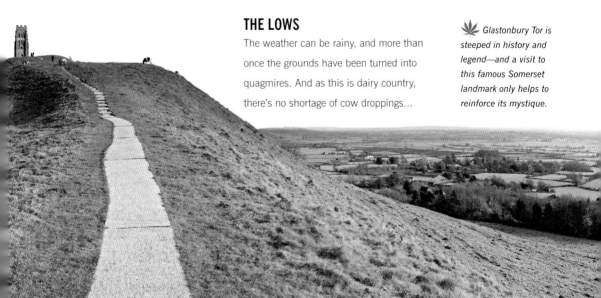

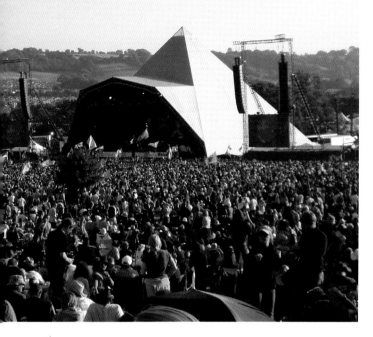

Glastonbury's unmistakable Pyramid Stage has featured an eclectic mix of acts, from US rapper Jay-Z to Welsh crooner Tom Jones—anything goes.

THE DOPE

Britain was once a world leader in industrial-hemp production, but the UK has only recently got into high-quality cannabis cultivation—and this overwhelmingly indoors. Until ten years ago, the cannabis product available in the British Isles was mostly hashish imported from Morocco and the Middle East. But more and more Brit growers have been emulating the example of the Netherlands across the North Sea, and many of the same strains available there can now be grown and partaken of in the UK—if perhaps not as openly or as cheaply.

THE FESTIVAL

Glastonbury has become a massive cultural event in the UK, with wide TV and radio coverage. The main stage—known as the "Pyramid Stage"—is on the north of the site;

the "Other Stage" is on the opposite side. In between there are tents featuring acoustic music, comedy acts, and a circus. There are activist, alternative-energy, and holistic-medicine exhibits in the Green Futures/Healing Fields area.

Since 1981, the festival has been organized by local farmer and site owner Michael Eavis, although his daughter Emily is gradually taking over. A portion of all the proceeds are donated to charities and political causes—recently Greenpeace and Oxfam have been beneficiaries. In the 1980s, there were some legal conflicts over the permits, and in 1990 there was an ugly outbreak of violence between New Age Travelers and security guards. In recent years the festival has gone more smoothly, however, and it is now unquestionably included in the UK's cultural calendar by the authorities and the public alike, drawing weekend revelers, hardcore "travelers," hippie grannies, and inner-city youth.

As a reflection of this diversity, the acts booked have moved on from the more rock/hippie roots of the event, and performers come from all over the world to play. Acts as wide ranging as Bob Dylan, Paul McCartney, Fairport Convention, The Who, Aswad, Van Morrison, Curtis Mayfield, the Smiths, Elvis Costello, the Pixies, the Orb, Lenny Kravitz, the Velvet Underground, REM, Radiohead,

Björk, Moby, White Stripes, Isaac Hayes, Sinead O'Connor, Coldplay, De La Soul, James Brown, Toots and the Maytals, Leonard Cohen, and Neil Diamond are just a few of the names to have graced the main stage. In 2008, there was also a degree of controversy when Jay-Z, the festival's first big rap booking, headlined, although his appearance turned out to be a triumph.

KNOW THE LAW

Festival organizers do not condone drug use onsite. The local police stress that they have a zero-tolerance approach to drugs in and around the festival site and that they will apply UK law to the letter. Although the UK has been moving toward a more lenient cannabis policy in recent years, the 2004 downgrading of cannabis classification from Class B to C was reversed in 2009. While possession of small quantities may be treated with a degree of leniency for adults, larger amounts and dealing and cultivation are likely to bring the full weight of the law down.

Dope Sheet

THE PRODUCT: Lack of reliable sunshine meant that, in the past, most cannabis had to be imported into the UK. More recently there is an increasing number of small-scale growers producing indoor varieties. Dealing at the festival is covert and illegal.

LOOK OUT FOR: Weird and wonderful alternative acts; an enormous variety of food stalls; if the sun's shining—a very happy, chilled-out atmosphere.

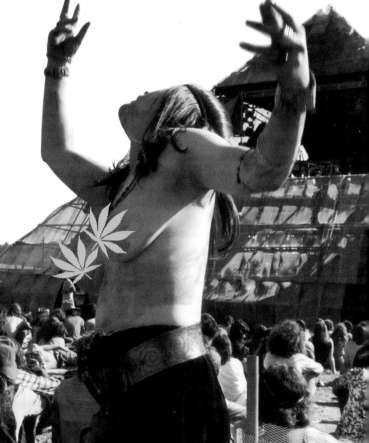

Glastonbury has been running pretty much annually for around 40 years.

HUMBOLDT REGGAE FESTIVALS USA

Northern California's Humboldt County is virtually synonymous with two of the Earth's most impressive varieties of flora: the giant redwoods— some specimens two or more millennia old—and the famous Emerald Triangle sinsemilla.

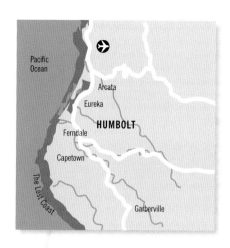

H umboldt is the heart of the dope-growing triangle that also includes Mendocino County down the coast to the south and Trinity County inland to the east. By a larger definition it also extends into Lake County that straddles the Coast Range in the south and Shasta County on the far slopes of the Trinity Alps to the east.

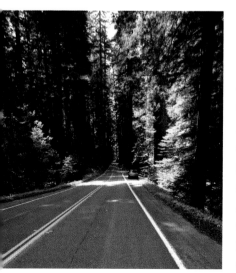

Giant Sequoias can live for hundreds and even thousands of years. The tallest examples can reach a height of over 265 feet (80 meters).

THE HIGHS

Arcata, on the north end of Humboldt Bay, is the county's center of hippie culture. It is also a great jumping-off point for excursions around the green, rugged, scenic county, including: the Avenue of the Giants through Humboldt Redwoods State Park; the Lost Coast national conservation area, with pine-clad mountains overlooking the sea; and Redwood National Park, which shelters more of the small fraction of surviving old-growth redwood forest. Nearer town you can check out redwoods at the Arcata Community Forest and adjacent Redwood Park. A more remote redwood expedition is to Headwaters Forest Reserve, which in 1999 was bought from the Pacific Lumber company by the state and federal government following a long campaign by Earth First! and allied groups, whose activists occupied the tree-tops to stave off the chain-saws. Access to the reserve must be arranged through the Arcata office of the US Bureau of Land Management.

Arcata also holds a 420 Festival—a public cannabis smoke-in every April 20 in the city's Redwood Park. In Laytonville is Area 101, which holds its own Mendocino Medical Marijuana Emerald Cup, where local strains—grown by producers affiliated with the Mendocino Medical Marijuana Advisory Board—are judged every December.

Heading inland from Humboldt into Trinity County on Highway 299, you leave behind the redwoods for Douglas fir, and the crunchy-granola hippie culture of the coast for a taste of the Old West. Your last stop before leaving Humboldt County is the Bigfoot Country Museum at Willow Creek. The somewhat precarious road follows the Trinity River, which plunges down from the Trinity Alps in some of California's most remote territory. There are still outlaw gold miners in the hills—as well as lots of dope growers.

THE LOWS

The Emerald Triangle's Wild West legacy is also alive in some negative ways. Growers—especially those who do it outlaw-style on public lands—have a reputation for booby-trapping their patches and guarding them with rifles. When hiking in the National Forests it is best to stick to the trail. This

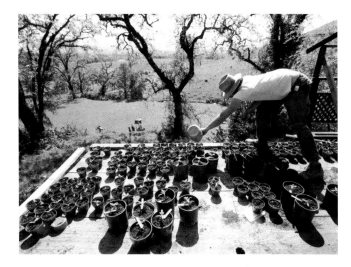

atmosphere has worsened in recent years as Mexican and Russian mafias have started to get into the local growing game, elbowing in on the hippies and mountain men.

The joint state–federal Campaign Against Marijuana Planting (CAMP) fills the skies with helicopters in the weeks leading up to the October harvest, and the California Highway Patrol maintains an aggressive presence on Highway 101 between Humboldt and San Francisco during harvest season.

Northern California has a long association with marijuana cultivation. Here a farmer from Gaberville fertilizes saplings. The potential profits have encouraged mafia gangs to move into production.

The tranquil Eel River is home to both Reggae Rising and Reggae on the River festivals.

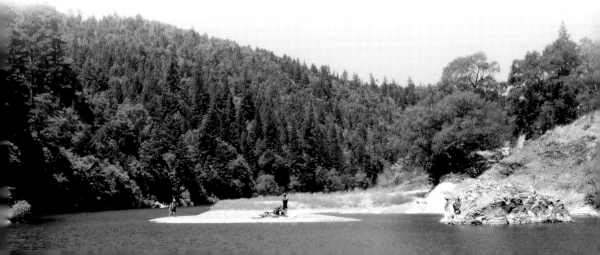

THE DOPE

Humboldt County has been a key incubator for high-potency cannabis strains. When the hippies first started growing there in the early 1970s, they used sativa seeds that they saved from the Mexican they'd been smoking. Later, some journeyed to Afghanistan to bring back more potent indica strains. The indica-sativa hybrid became the emblematic local sinsemilla. Twenty years ago, indica-heavy "Kush" strains were all the rage—named for Afghanistan's Hindu Kush mountains. The most popular was the legendary Skunk. These strains notoriously induced a "heavy," somatic kind of high, as opposed to the "lighter," more cerebral sativa buzz. Kush and Skunk have become something of a Holy Grail, as they have largely been re-hybridized into less crushingly potent strains.

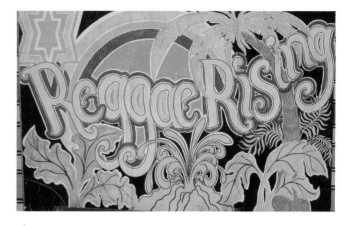

A mural publicizing the Reggae Rising festival, where top reggae acts from around the world perform.

Although not a cannabis event, festival goers to Reggae Rising know how to party.

THE FESTIVALS

The three-day Reggae Rising Music Festival has been held every July or August since 2007 at Dimmick Ranch, situated on a picturesque turn of the Eel River outside Piercy—just below Garberville off Highway 101 and just above the Humboldt–Mendocino line. It is not a cannabis festival in any explicit sense, but it draws world-class reggae talent, including UB40, Junior Reed, the Original Wailers, Queen Ifrica, Rootz Underground, Toots and The Maytals, and Aswad. There is a live video feed from the stage on three large viewing screens.

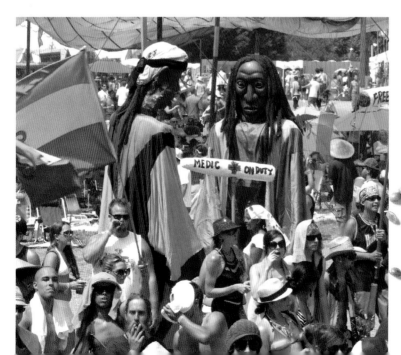

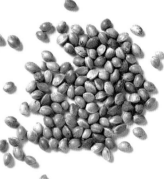

For those holding "VIP tickets," there is shaded seating, wine-tasting, hors d'oeuvres, and massages. For everyone, there are craft booths, food vendors, and a special children's area called Kidlandia. Even after the main stage shuts down, DJs at the South Beach Dome keep the party going till dawn.

Reggae Rising has its roots in the Reggae on the River Festival, which began more than twenty years ago as a fundraising concert to rebuild the Mateel Community Center in Redway after it was burned down by an arsonist in 1984. However, disagreements between the Mateel Community Center and the promoter and landowner led to two separate festivals, and now Reggae on the River continues as an annual one-day fundraiser for the Mateel Center at Benbow Lake State Park (also on the Eel River) a few weeks earlier in July. It also draws top talent, featuring acts such as the Abyssinians, Queen Omega, and the Mighty Diamonds.

KNOW THE LAW

Cannabis has been decriminalized in California since 1975. Although possession of even small quantities should, by law, incur a fine, it is often not enforced. Larger amounts, however, are more likely to lead to a fine or even prison, and cultivation and dealing on any scale will certainly get the offender into serious trouble. The Compassionate Use Act of 1996 effectively legalized cannabis grown or consumed for medical purposes, although the feds do not recognize California's medical-marijuana law, and state authorities have not always been supportive of medical-cannabis providers busted by the DEA.

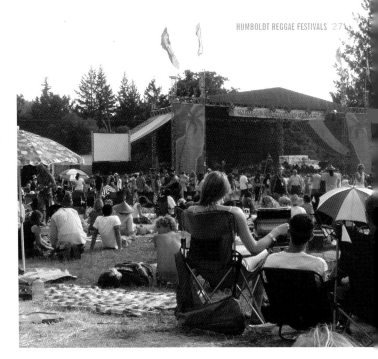

In 2009, Reggae on the River celebrated its 25th anniversary and the festival is still raising money for the Mateel Community Center.

Dope Sheet

THE PRODUCT: Well-established indica-heavy sinsemilla is widely found.

LOOK OUT FOR: The Kinetic Sculpture Race from Arcata to Ferndale occurs each Memorial Day weekend; Arcata hosts a public cannabis "smoke-in," a 420 Festival every April 20; Humboldt in general has some good hiking trails through a number of state and national parks.

CANNABIS CUP
THE NETHERLANDS

At *High Times* magazine's annual Cannabis Cup in Amsterdam, judges spend several days visiting some of the many cannabis-friendly "coffeeshops" that dot the city, sampling a wide variety of strains from all over the world.

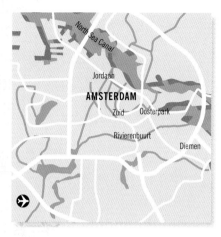

They peer through magnifying glasses and even microscopes to examine the resin exuding from the glands at the tops of the flowering female plants. They smoke cannabis in cigarette form and from half a dozen types of pipes developed for the connoisseur. They eat cannabis cakes and cannabis bon-bons covered in Holland's finest chocolate. They discuss the pros and cons of many varieties. They debate the relative merits of marijuana grown in soil and hydroponic marijuana (grown in rockwool or sponge using nutrient-rich water). Finally, they vote on which varieties combine the subtleties of taste, color, aroma, and psychophysical effect that mark a championship strain.

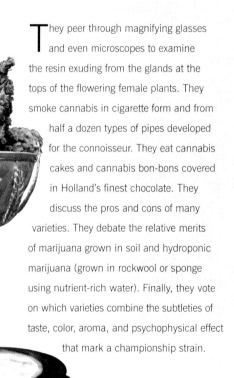

The High Times *Cannabis Cup is awarded annually to the winner of the Best Overall Cannabis category.*

THE FESTIVAL

The Cannabis Cup—held over five days during November—was launched in 1987 by Steven Hager, Creative Director of *High Times*. "Here what we do is not criminal," Hager told the magazine. "No one is threatening to forfeit homes for growing half a dozen plants to use as medicine for glaucoma or muscular sclerosis, or threatening to take our children if we are caught smoking a joint. Here in Amsterdam we can walk into a coffeeshop and see a menu that includes not only sandwiches but a daily selection of marijuana and hashish."

While the early events were private affairs between the editors of *High Times* and a handful of Dutch growers and coffeeshop owners, the Cup quickly grew. By 1991, several rock musicians as well as Dr. Erik Fromberg of the Netherlands National Institute of Alcohol and Drugs asked to join in the judging. In 1993, when the event was opened to the public for the first time, nearly a hundred judges served. Today, it's been claimed that around 2,000 members of the public purchase official judging credentials, and many more from around the world attend.

The Cup does not provide judges with the cannabis samples. These must be purchased at the coffeeshops—although many shops have booths at the expo and openly ply judges with samples of their product. A winning strain translates into prestige and profit for Amsterdam's purveyors.

The different award categories can vary. In the past the awards have included Best Overall Cannabis, Best Hydroponically Grown Cannabis, Best Bioponically Grown Cannabis, and Best "Nederhash" (domestic Netherlands hashish). There are also awards for cannabis freedom fighters. Tom Forçade, the late founder of *High Times*, was inducted into the Counterculture Hall of Fame in 2009.

In recent years, the expo has been held in Amsterdam's PowerZone venue, with nightly concerts at the Melkweg nightclub. Entertainment is provided by New York's permier reggae act, the Cannabis Cup Band, and other headliners have included Rita Marley, Steel Pulse, Bushman, Andrew Tosh, Redman, Jefferson Starship, the Patti Smith Group, Tommy Chong of the famed Cheech and Chong hippie comedy act, and Native American shaman-poet John Trudell.

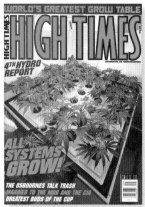

High Times, sponsors of the Cup, has been promoting the legalization of cannabis since the magazine was founded in 1974.

Amsterdam attracts over four million visitors each year.

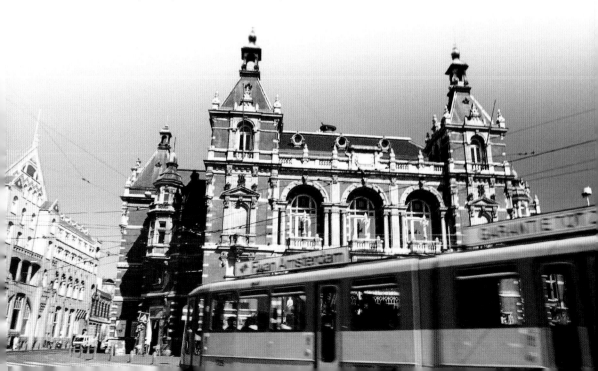

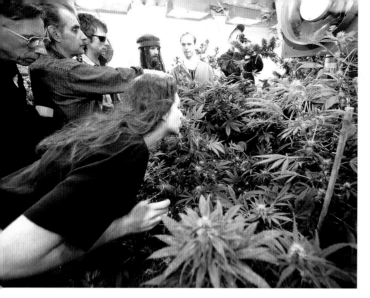

as Know Good Buds, or KGB), run by Americans who served prison time for growing marijuana and then relocated to the Netherlands so they could grow in peace.

DAY TRIPPING

In addition to the expo, the seminars, and coffeeshop hopping, there are a number of side trips available to the visitors as well—champagne boat rides on the city's canals; visits to indoor grow-rooms; and a tour of the Hash Museum in Amsterdam's red-light district, devoted to the historical uses of hemp and the ancient tradition of hashish smoking around the world.

One of the most exciting day trips is a tour of Cannabis Castle—an old Victorian mansion near Rotterdam, where for more than a decade the Sensi Seed Company has been breeding new strains. The castle staff dress up for visitors in old Dutch costumes and powdered wigs; antique castle furnishings are reupholstered in hemp. Owner Ben Dronkers and his longtime collaborator, genetic whizz Nevil Schoenbottom, have turned the castle into one of the world's most important repositories of cannabis strains—drawn from every region in which the plant has been cultivated. A tour of Cannabis Castle usually includes a visit to the underground network of grow-rooms where their hybrid seed strains are developed.

🌿 Visitors inspecting plants at Cannabis Castle, a mansion around 40 miles (60 kilometers) outside of Amsterdam. Some of the plants are over twenty years old.

Attractions around town include Positronics Salon, a store that specializes in indoor gardening equipment and gives lessons in hashish making; the Green House Coffeeshop, run by multiple winner Arjan; Barney's Uptown, a smoke-friendly restaurant; and the specialty seed house Cannabis in Amsterdam (CIA—also known

🌿 Derry, the proprietor of Barney's coffeeshop, accepting the Cannabis Cup in 2004.

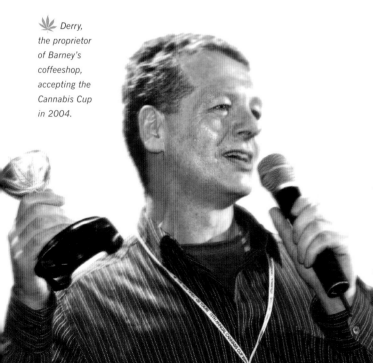

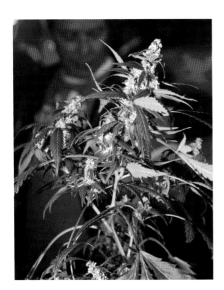

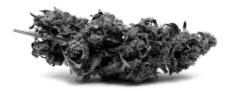 A plant at the Paradise Seeds stand at the 2008 Cannabis Cup Expo.

The Sensi Seed Bank's 1994 winning strain, Jack Herer, was named for the American guru of the hemp movement, who spent more than twenty years uncovering a mountain of US government material about the plant's benefits that was buried after cannabis was made illegal in 1937. The fruit of this effort, his book *The Emperor Wears No Clothes*, has become an underground classic.

For more details on the highs, lows, and laws of the Netherlands, see our Amsterdam entry in the following section (see page 58).

Cannabis Cup winners to date

1988 - Skunk #1 from Cultivator's Choice

1989 - Early Pearl/Skunk #1 x Northern Lights #5/Haze from the Seed Bank

1990 - Northern Lights #5 from the Seed Bank

1991 - Skunk from Free City

1992 - Haze x Skunk #1 from Homegrown Fantasy

1993 - Haze x Northern Lights #5 from Sensi Seed Bank

1994 - Jack Herer from Sensi Seed Bank

1995 - White Widow from the Green House

1996 - White Russian from De Dampkring

1997 - Peace Maker from De Dampkring

1998 - Super Silver Haze from the Green House

1999 - Super Silver Haze from the Green House

2000 - Blueberry from the Noon

2001 - Sweet Tooth from Barney's

2002 - Morning Glory from Barney's

2003 - Hawaiian Snow from the Green House

2004 - Amnesia Haze from Barney's

2005 - Willie Nelson from Barney's

2006 - Arjan's Ultra Haze #1 from the Green House

2007 - G-13 Haze from Barney's

2008 - Super Lemon Haze from the Green House

2009 - Super Lemon Haze from the Green House

TORONTO FREEDOM FESTIVAL CANADA

Canada's most populous and cosmopolitan city hosts the country's biggest cannabis festival. It also has a cannabis-themed district, which is (more or less) tolerated by the local authorities: Yongesterdam—a play on Amsterdam.

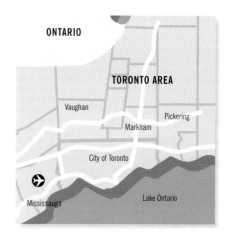

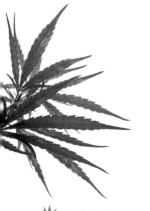

🍁 Located on the shores of Lake Ontario, Toronto is a cosmopolitan city, with its own Little Italy, Little Korea, and no less than six Chinatowns.

This aspiring "green-light district" (located on the 600 block of Yonge Street) was launched in 1994 with the opening of the Toronto Hemp Company (THC—get it?) at 665 Yonge. A few allied businesses have since sprung up in the vicinity, with the Yongesterdam area starting to rival Vancouver as the foremost Canadian cannabis scene.

THE HIGHS

Billing itself as the "World's Largest and Greatest Hemp Store/Cannabis Culture Shop," THC boasts a wide variety of hemp clothing, cosmetics, fabric, food, and paper products as well as vaporizers, rolling papers, and the like. Nearby is the KindRed Café, around the corner at 7 Breadalbane Street, Toronto's Green Bean Coffee House, specializing in fair-trade, organic, fresh-roasted coffees, teas, and munchies. (Members of the KindRed Café club also gain access to the "smoke-friendly patio.") At 667 Yonge is Vapor Central, "Toronto's Vapor Shop and Comparison Lounge," featuring such new technologies the Herbal Aire vaporizer, "which allows you to inhale the medicinal goodness of your favorite herb without the harmful effects of smoking." Next is Sacred

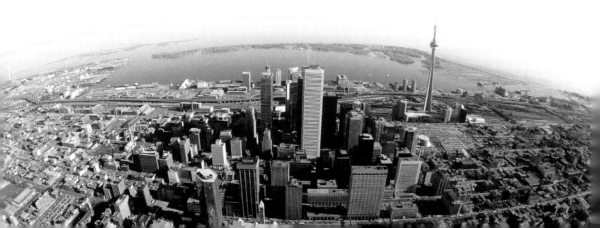

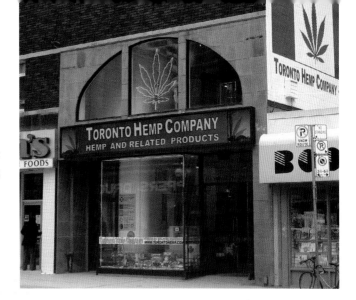

Seed, at 2A Dundonald Street (also just off Yonge), 'Toronto's exotic seed and house-plant shop', with an unbelievably diverse collection of medicinal and horticultural plant seeds from all over the world as well as living plants, dried herbs and related products. Then comes Toronto Art Glass, at 28 Dundonald, with live glass-blowing demos.

Yonge Street is one of downtown Toronto's main drags, so Yongesterdam is a good jumping-off point to explore the rest of the city including Toronto's six Chinatowns. The oldest and most central of these extends north, south and east from the corner of Spadina Avenue and Dundas Street – starting several streets west of Yonge. It's teeming with restaurants and markets, offering Vietnamese and other Asian fare as well as Chinese – a great place to try curried eel or snail vermicelli. There are all kinds of specialist shops, many selling traditional Chinese herbal remedies.

To the west, between College and Dundas streets, is Kensington Market – which has the best claim to being Toronto's bohemian enclave. A little on the run-down side, it is home to lots of vintage clothing shops and shops selling food from all over the world. On College, between Bathurst and Ossington, is Toronto's Little Italy, with plenty of eateries. It has also got one of the city's most vibrant summer nightlife scenes, with many bars

opening their patios into the small hours. Little Korea is centred on Bathurst and Bloor to the north; a second Koreatown has also sprung up near the North York district back on Yonge Street, completing our circle.

THE LOWS

Gentrification has taken its toll on Toronto. Yorkville, not far from Yongesterdam, used to be the city's bohemian cultural quarter. In the past it was the matrix of some of Canada's most celebrated musical personalities such as Joni Mitchell and Neil Young, and by the late 1960s it was the Canadian capital of the hippy movement. Following the gentrification of recent years, however, it has become an upscale domain of high-end art galleries, fashion boutiques, antique shops and the like. If you've got the bread, enjoy it – but it ain't what it was.

The Toronto Hemp Company sells just about every hemp-related product available. The shop is also a resource centre providing information on every aspect of cannabis and cannabis production.

The intersection of Yonge and Breadalbane – you're in the right area for a whole host of cannabis-related businesses.

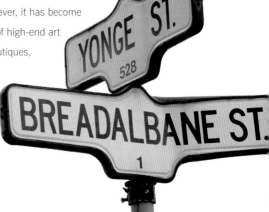

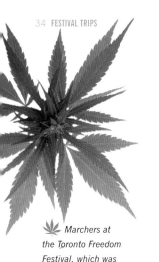

🌿 Marchers at the Toronto Freedom Festival, which was first held in 2007.

For all its cultural diversity, and despite its seedy sections, Toronto can seem a little sterile at first. The city's poet laureate, Pier Giorgio Di Cicco, famously said: "Toronto is a city that has yet to fall in love with itself." Other Canadians complain about the high rents, dirty air and beaches, and the attitude of the locals. However, by the standards of, say, New York City, the people are actually very friendly and polite, and by the standards of Los Angeles, the air is pretty clean.

THE DOPE

Ontario outdoor strains of varying quality start showing up around October—local hydroponic is high-quality and available year-round, of course. BC Hydro is also available, usually at a slightly higher price and potency. Organic sinsemilla is also popular.

Cannabis is quite widely available. One source who picked up some bud (a local strain dubbed Golden Harvest) not far from Yongesterdam reported: "Just look for the pizza shop that sells no pizzas."

THE FESTIVAL

The Toronto Freedom Festival has been held in early May since 2007 at the city's Queen's Park North. The Freedom Festival presents multiple stages featuring local roots, rock, funk, and hip-hop talent, as well as a vast array of vendors, artists, and exhibits. Numerous activist groups have tables and displays on human rights, environmental issues, and alternative medicines. Some 12,000 attended in 2009. An estimated

5,000 also participated that day in a march to decriminalize cannabis, coordinated with the Global Marijuana March campaign.

Back at the park, the cannabis-themed carnival offered onstage poetry slams, local and international DJ and electronica talent, 25 multiethnic food vendors, and a Freedom Film Festival at the park's theater. *High Times* magazine had its own Vendors' Village, showcasing cannabis culture from around the world. The local Toronto group CALM (Cannabis as Living Medicine) hosted a Medicinal Marijuana Pavilion, offering information on medicating with cannabis and patients' rights under Ontario and Canadian law.

The organizers say that the fundamental principle behind the Toronto Freedom Festival is free choice. "A person's choice may not be the same as ours but their freedom to choose should be," says festival cofounder The Gerbz. "Toronto is happy to lead the way for the Global Marijuana March."

KNOW THE LAW

Cannabis possession is illegal throughout Canada, although there is a large degree of de facto tolerance in British Columbia, which some in Ontario would like to emulate. However, Freedom Festival organizers boast that nobody has ever been arrested at their event, which is a good sign.

Dope Sheet

THE PRODUCT: BC Bud provides the best available high-quality hydroponic, but also available are locally grown outdoor strains, hydroponic, and organic sinsemilla.

LOOK OUT FOR: A multicultural atmosphere; summer in particular sees a lively bar and restaurant scene; Kensington Market for laid-back bohemia; Lake Ontario has beaches, water sports, bike trails, etc.

Officially, possession of small amounts for personal use can lead to a prison sentence, although this is unlikely to be enforced. Prison is, however, more likely for dealing or cultivation. Meanwhile, activists are supporting Bill C-359 in Ottawa, which would decriminalize across Canada.

Marc Emery addresses the audience at the festival. Emery sold cannabis seeds via a mail order company, some of which made their way across the border. He is now facing extradition to the US.

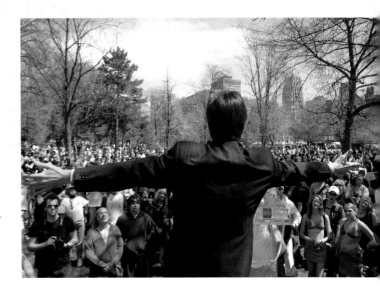

THE GREAT MIDWEST MARIJUANA HARVEST FESTIVAL USA

The biggest and oldest cannabis festival in the Midwest is, naturally enough, held in the region's most open-minded town and the capital of its most forward-looking state.

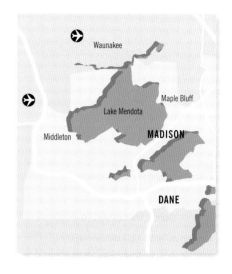

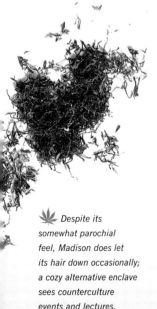

Despite its somewhat parochial feel, Madison does let its hair down occasionally; a cozy alternative enclave sees counterculture events and lectures.

Despite the Midwest's current conservative reputation, it was the heartland of the Populist and Progressive movements of the late 19th and early 20th centuries which sought to restrict the power of corporations and support small farmers. The Progressive standard-bearer Robert La Follette was Wisconsin's governor from 1901 to 1906 and then a US senator until his death in 1925. The legacy of the Populist and Progressive movements is alive and well in contemporary Madison, and today lots of struggling farmers are turning from growing corn to cannabis to stay profitable.

THE HIGHS

The home of the flagship University of Wisconsin campus, Madison is the Midwest's haven of alternative culture, with food cooperatives, great mountain-bike trails through the scenic lakelands to the west of town, and a strong ecological consciousness.

The Williamson Street neighborhood, starting around nine blocks east of the high-domed State Capitol building, the city's central hub, is Madison's alternative enclave, with plenty of coffeeshops to visit. One, the Escape Java Joint and Gallery (940 Williamson), hosts the monthly meeting of Madison's National

Organization for the Reform of Marijuana Laws (NORML) chapter as well as frequent events and lectures sponsored by the group. The Madison Infoshop, another key activist check-in point, is just a block away from here at 1019 Williamson.

Also in this neighborhood—which is actually a little land bridge between two of Madison's four lakes, Mendota and Monona—are the Hempen Goods store at 911 Williamson and Fat Pinky Glass, a glassblowers, at 951 Williamson, which has some truly amazing creations, including glass jewelry and art pieces as well as pipes.

The first weekend in May, Madison hosts the Mifflin Street Block Party, a bacchanalia that has its roots in a 1969 anti-war street party that exploded into a riot when it was attacked by the police. Today it is characterized by live music, poetry slams, and massive beer consumption. The same folks who organize the Harvest Festival also stage a Pot Parade to coincide with the Block Party. The parade, generally drawing a few hundred, is Madison's contribution to the worldwide Global Marijuana March, and witnesses report that joints are thrown out to the crowd en masse.

The region around Madison is of special interest to chroniclers of hemp history. Throughout the 1920s, the US Department of Agriculture ran its Wisconsin Agriculture Experiment Station at Arlington, 3 miles (5 kilometers) north of Madison, where researcher Andrew Wright carried out investigations into the industrial applications of the hemp plant. Wright made his home at Viroqua, about 75 miles (120 kilometers) northwest of Madison, where the state's leading hemp researcher, Dr. David West, is today collecting an archive on Wisconsin's industrial-hemp legacy.

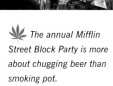

The annual Mifflin Street Block Party is more about chugging beer than smoking pot.

THE LOWS

Madison is a pleasant enough place but it's a little sleepy and provincial by big-city standards—and it goes to bed early. It also has little in the way of cultural diversity— the city is 90 percent white. The winters are notoriously long and harsh so unless you are into cross-country skiing or other winter sports, avoid the area between November and March.

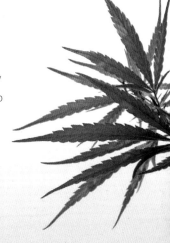

Dope Sheet

🌿 **THE PRODUCT:** Outdoor-grown Northern Lights strain available end of September; indoor-grown is available throughout the year, but expensive. Stay clear of the wild "Ditchweed."

🌿 **LOOK OUT FOR:** A very green-friendly, ecologically minded town; farmers' cooperatives; lakeside mountain-bike trails; Williamson Street neighborhood has much to recommend it for those seeking interesting and alternative stores.

Wisconsin's outdoor commercial crop comes in at the end of September, and the best of it rates with that of Northern California. Although today associated with the hothouses of Amsterdam, local Wisconsin growers actually developed the famous Northern Lights strain as an outdoor variety adapted to the state's short growing season. "The trick is to get it to flower early," says one source. "Only the ones that start ripening by September 1 make any sense here." In the 1970s, an indica brought back from Afghanistan was all the rage with Wisconsin growers, resulting in the local product known colloquially as "Wisghani." This has today been hybridized with other strains, and the original Wisghani probably no longer exists.

THE DOPE

"Ditchweed"—a feral descendant of the industrial hemp that was cultivated in the state before World War II—abounds in Wisconsin, despite relentlessly quixotic efforts by authorities to eradicate it. However, smokers would have to toke an awful lot of this stuff to catch the slightest buzz.

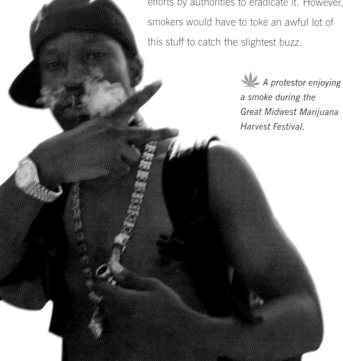

🌿 *A protestor enjoying a smoke during the Great Midwest Marijuana Harvest Festival.*

Both local and out-of-state, mostly West Coast, indoor is available year-round in Wisonsin, but it is pretty expensive.

THE FESTIVAL

The Great Midwest Marijuana Harvest Festival has been held in downtown Madison every first weekend in October since 1970, drawing up to 15,000 in recent years. The Harvest Fest is sponsored by Madison NORML, Wisconsin NORML, the university chapter of Students for Sensible Drug Policy (SSDP), the Wisconsin Hemp Order, and Is My Medicine Legal Yet? (IMMLY). The Wisconsin Hemp Order is the recent revival of the state hemp-growers' union launched in

1917. IMMLY is a reference to a wheelchair-bound sufferer of the debilitating Ehlers-Danlos Syndrome, Jacki Rickert, who was apparently promised by Bill Clinton on a Madison campaign stop in 1992 that she would have legal access to medicinal cannabis. She is still waiting.

Live music at the Harvest Fest in recent years has included jam-band Baghdad Scuba Review, beer-rockers BUrP, and the electric folk of the Reverend Eddie Danger. Speakers have included Jacki Rickert, local organizer Ben Masel (a perennial candidate for public office on a pro-hemp line), and Kentucky hemp crusader Gatewood Galbraith.

With police generally drawn by a Big Ten football match that weekend, tokers at the Harvest Fest have thus far been able to smoke unmolested.

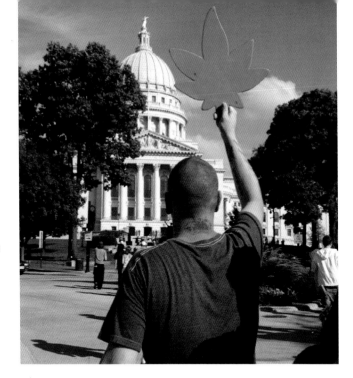

Madison Harvest Festival marchers protesting and lobbying at the Capitol.

KNOW THE LAW

Possession of marijuana in Wisconsin is technically punishable by a six-month prison sentence, doubled for second convictions. However, Madison passed a decriminalization ordinance in 1976. State law didn't change, but the state legislature passed an opt-out provision leaving it up to the discretion of the local district attorney whether to bring charges under Wisconsin law or the more lenient local ordinance—and the Madison DA has had a blanket policy of using the local ordinance.

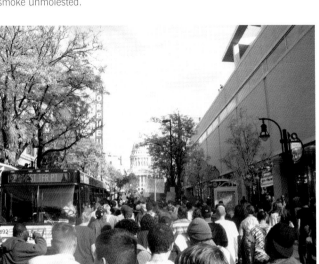

Along with marching and protesting, the Harvest Fest features guest speakers and an array of bands.

NIMBIN MARDI GRASS AUSTRALIA

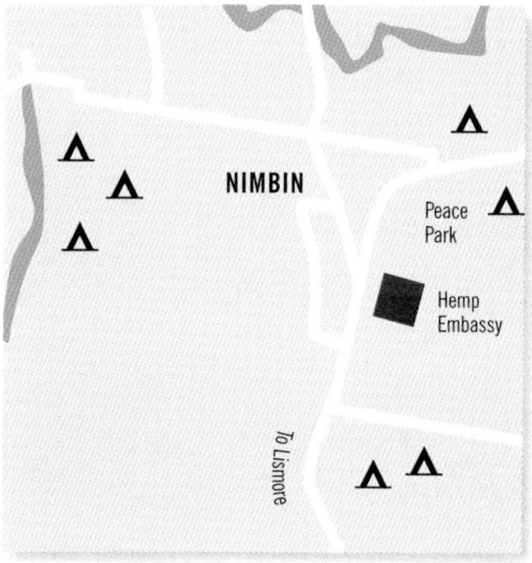

On the foothills of an extinct volcano inland from scenic Cape Byron in New South Wales, the village of Nimbin is the heart of Australia's "Rainbow Region"—a center of back-to-the-land hippie culture and cannabis cultivation.

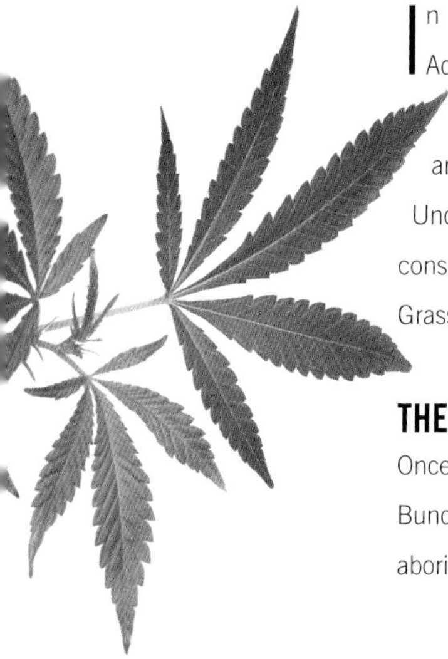

NIMBIN
Peace Park
Hemp Embassy
To Lismore

In 1973, the village hosted an Age of Aquarius festival, which brought the first wave of long-haired settlers to Nimbin and established its reputation as Down Under's rural heartland of alternative consciousness. Since 1993, the Mardi Grass festival has been an annual event.

THE HIGHS

Once a sacred initiation site for the Bundjalung tribe of the local Kooris— aboriginals of southeastern Australia—

Nimbin was only settled by Europeans in the late 19th century. There was little there when the hippies started arriving in the early 1970s, so the cannabis culture is deeply ingrained. The town hosts a Hemp Embassy (information center and activist check-in point), Hemp Bar (a coffeeshop, where smoking was encouraged until the authorities cracked down on it a few years back), and Nimbin Museum (sporting the works of local alterno-artists and craftsmen). There are plenty of other psychedelic-tinged cafés and craft shops.

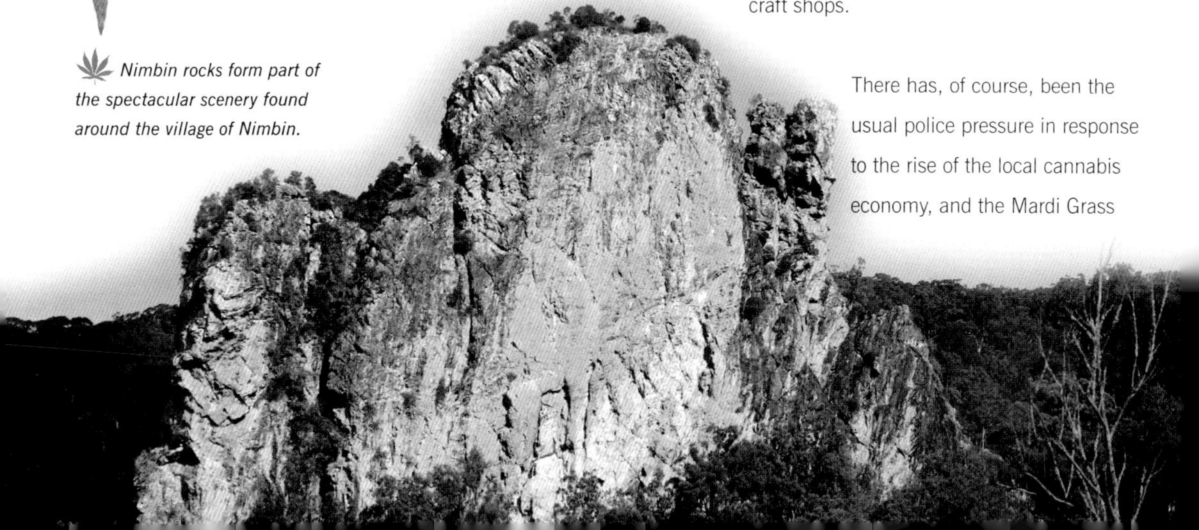

There has, of course, been the usual police pressure in response to the rise of the local cannabis economy, and the Mardi Grass

Nimbin rocks form part of the spectacular scenery found around the village of Nimbin.

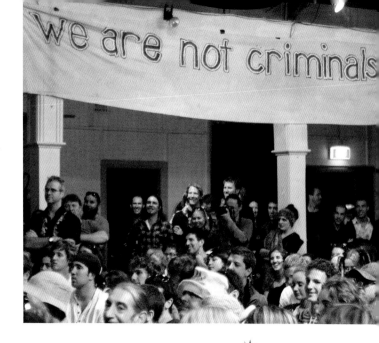

festival grew out of efforts to protest against—and even directly resist—the heavy-handed enforcement. In one famous escapade in January 1997, activists actually chained themselves to police helicopters when they were parked outside a motel for the night. The pilots awoke to find their birds surrounded by hippies and the press. The embarrassment put an end to the anti-cannabis overflights—for a while.

Despite its notoriety, Nimbin is small and a little hard to find. It is around 110 miles (180 kilometers) south of Brisbane, on the slopes of the Great Dividing Range. You can't get a bus directly to the village from any major city, but there is a local line that connects it to Lismore town 20 miles (30 kilometers) to the south. Nimbin has a few bed-and-breakfasts, hostels, and small hotels, as well as campgrounds.

There's some spectacular scenery around the town. A recommended day trip for nature lovers is to the nearby Nightcap National Park, which protects the caldera of Mount Warning volcano, its rugged inclines clad in subtropical rainforest, with waterfalls and lush green gullies.

THE LOWS

In addition to the aforementioned police pressure (which escalates during the April–June harvest season), Nimbin unfortunately has a persistent problem with heroin use, which has raised the undercurrent of paranoia. Especially during Mardi Grass, there is heavy policing on all roads in and out of town. Attendees should be prepared to have car and body searched, and possibly submit to drug and alcohol checks via saliva swab. There have been a number of drug arrests at the festival over the years.

Nimbin was in the middle of rainforest until the settlers cleared it a century ago, and many of the Mardi Grass festivals have been wet. In 1996 the rain was so heavy that the village was virtually cut off—so festival-goers should take their rain gear.

🌿 *The purpose of the first festival was to encourage peaceful protest against heavy-handed police activity.*

🌿 *Police presence is historically conspicuous at Mardi Grass.*

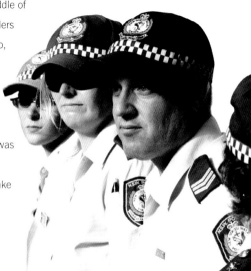

🌿 *A man hands out loose joints during Nimbin's antiprohibition Mardi Grass festival.*

THE DOPE

Local cultivators produce the same kinds of sativa-indica hybrids as their counterparts in Hawaii and Northern California, with some of the locally developed strains including Rainbow Dreaming, Bubbleberry (a cross between the "bubbly," sativa-heavy Bubblegum and the fruity-fragrant Blueberry), Jack Flash, and Bushman. Cannabis tends to be somewhat cheaper in Australia than in the US and Europe.

THE FESTIVAL

Despite the play on "Mardi Gras," Nimbin Mardi Grass isn't held in February but the first weekend of May—the height of Australia's cannabis harvest season. Thousands descend on the village for the annual celebration of local cannabis culture. In addition to nightly live music at the Harvest Ball and Picker's Ball, there's a Nimbin Cannabis Cup, where

🌿 *A competitor at work during the Hemp Olympix. Training is undertaken throughout the year.*

local strains are judged, and a Prohibition Protest Rally, in which the gaily clad Ganja Faeries parade through town toting a giant float in the shape of a joint (sheets stitched together over a bamboo frame) adorned with the official Mardi Grass slogan: "Let It Grow!"

Among the sillier events is the Hemp Olympix, featuring competitions in a variety of joint-rolling disciplines (including speed rolling, rolling in adverse conditions, and rolling in the dark), the bong throw and yell, seed sorting, and, finally, the Grower's Iron Person (as opposed to Iron Man, of course) event, where runners must first carry a 44-pound (20-kilogram) sack of fertilizer, then a bucket of water, and, finally, harvested crop—a testament to the rigors faced by cannabis cultivators.

Mardi Grass has its origins in a March 1993 incident when a spontaneous protest erupted after a wave of police raids, arrests, and harassment. Locals marched on the police station, pelting it with eggs and toilet paper. Negative media accounts ensued, and Nimbin Hemp Embassy members decided to hold a peaceful protest in a nonconfrontational atmosphere on May 1. That was the first Mardi Grass, drawing over 1,000. The all-volunteer Mardi Grass Organizing Body (MOB) was formed and the resolution taken to hold a Mardi Grass every year until cannabis prohibition ends.

The event has grown bigger each year. Many attendees caravan to Nimbin for the festival from Byron Bay in a "Kombi Konvoy" of psychedelic-painted Volkswagen minibuses known as "combis." A full Mardi Grass pass can be bought that includes access to all events related to the festival, as well as two nights at a local campsite (tents not included).

KNOW THE LAW

South Australia, Western Australia, Northern Territory, and the Australian Capital Territory around Canberra have all decriminalized cannabis. Ironically, Queensland and New South Wales—the center of cannabis culture in Australia—have not; neither have Victoria or Tasmania. This means possession is a criminal offense throughout the eastern part the country—with the exception of

Canberra—where the bulk of the population live. Personal possession can incur a prison sentence, but this seems rarely to be enforced. Penalties are stiffer—and more often enforced—for dealing or growing. No Australian state currently has a medical-marijuana law on the books.

> ### Dope Sheet
> **THE PRODUCT:** Sativa-indica hybrids similar to those grown in Hawaii and California abound. Rainbow Dreaming, Bubbleberry, Jack Flash, and Bushman are particular strains.
>
> **LOOK OUT FOR:** Hemp Olympix; Harvest Ball and Picker's Ball; the "Kombi Konvoy" of psychedelic colored Combi minibuses; Nightcap National Park features stunning, subtropical rainforest scenery.

You won't be surprised that green is the predominant color during the Mardi Grass parade—as worn by these Ganja Faeries on their way to the Peace Park.

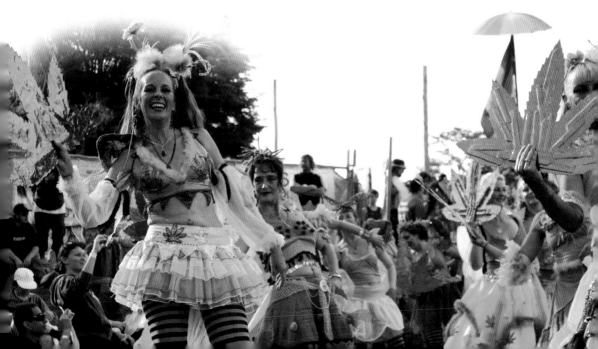

THE RAINBOW GATHERING USA

Every year since 1972, the Rainbow Family of Living Light has been holding its summer gathering in the National Forests of the USA, bouncing to a different state each year, from coast to coast.

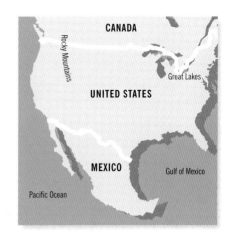

Rainbow People congregating in California during the Gathering of 2004.

A loose network of hippie tribes that celebrate their diversity, the Rainbow People caravan cross-country for the annual back-to-nature affair that starts building in June and climaxes with a silent meditation for world peace when the rest of the USA is setting off fireworks on July 4. These gatherings aspire to be temporary living alternatives to mass society and a working model of a world based on cooperation and giving rather than competition and money. There is an ethic of maximum freedom and tolerance, which extends to nudity, drug use, and all manner of uninhibited behavior.

THE HIGHS

The Rainbow Gathering is usually held in a place of outstanding natural beauty, with several camps scattered throughout the woods around a big central meadow where nightly councils, daily drum-circles and the July 4 meditation are convened. The camps—from just a cluster of tents to elaborate affairs with operating kitchens and rustic performance stages—are run by everything from long-haired Jesus freaks and Hare Krishnas to nomadic ecstasy-seekers ("bliss bunnies") and rasta-hippie hybrids;

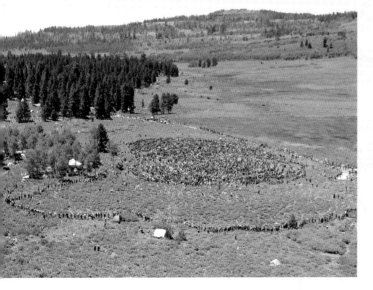

earthy rural homesteaders to grungy urban anarchists; middle-class weekend warriors to outright hobos.

The event is, by consensus, noncommercial, with no money exchanged on site, although a Magic Hat is passed around at the main circle for supply-run donations. There's no electricity and no port-o-sans. Unless you are a weekender who parachutes in for the big party on July 4, be prepared to put shovel to earth to dig a latrine and to pitch in on communal cooking. When you get to the site—generally there will be quite a trek from the offsite parking—there's a Welcome Home center with maps and information to get you oriented. Pack in your own food, and pack out your—nonbiodegradable—trash.

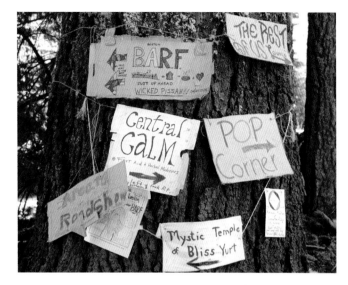

Health care at the gatherings is provided at the CALM (Center for Alternative Living Medicine) tent—reminiscent of a MASH tent—staffed by a loose coalition of licensed doctors, nurses, chiropractors, acupuncturists, holistic healers, homeopaths, and herbalists that grew out of the gatherings. There's also a Kiddie Village which provides childcare.

🌿 *The Rainbow Gatherings feature a mind-blowing array of alternative people and practices.*

🌿 *The gatherings emphasize community and cooperation, with a large dose of laissez-faire.*

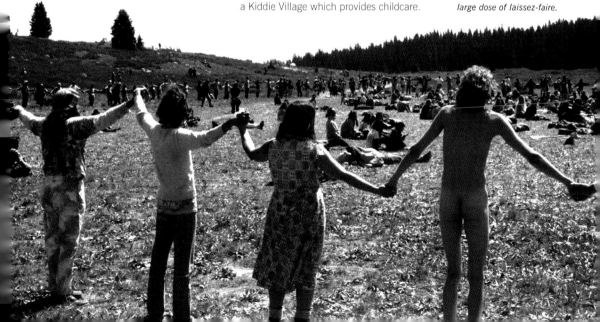

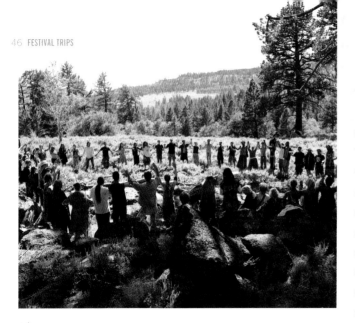

🌿 *Circles of silent meditation are central features of all Rainbow Gatherings.*

🌿 *People from all walks of life attend the gatherings, from spiritualists and hippies to weekend revelers.*

In addition to the summer national gathering, there are smaller regional gatherings held throughout the year around the USA, and a winter gathering is held most years in Florida's Ocala National Forest. The most hardcore Rainbow People drift from gathering to gathering throughout the year, but most of the local gatherings draw people from within the region. Other events are also organized in Europe (since 1983), and in 2006 a spring-equinox gathering was held in eastern Turkey, attended by people from all over the world and representing all major religions, denominations, and political affiliations in a spirit of common humanity. As Garrick Beck, a longtime member of the Rainbow Family, states: "They let their children play together, share each other's recipes. That's how we can get along. It's not a pie-in-the-sky routine; it's right here on earth. Sharing and caring is the essence of spirituality, the number-one lesson that is at the core of every religion."

THE LOWS

There have, predictably, been many problems with the authorities over the years—mostly relating to the legal right to gather. This has, on occasion, turned ugly, with some heavy-handed interference by the Forest Service police. However, in recent years the dialogue has been going better and, after some legal hassles, Rainbow organizers now seem to have arrived at an accommodation with federal authorities.

With up to 15,000 camped in one place, it is important to maintain awareness of hygiene. If you establish a camp, be careful to dig your latrine far away from water sources, although cases of the "Rainbow Runs" haven't been a serious problem in recent years.

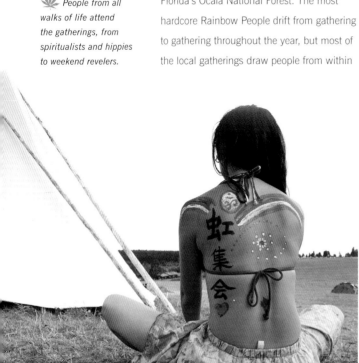

Dope Sheet

🍁 **THE PRODUCT:** Specific strains of cannabis will vary from location to location; natural psychedelics also feature heavily.

🍁 **LOOK OUT FOR:** Good old-fashioned naked hippies; healing areas; vast human circles of silent meditation.

THE DOPE

There is fairly open use of cannabis—and peyote, mushrooms, and other psychedelics. Organics are emphasized, and synthetic or processed drugs generally discouraged. Sharing is widespread—commercial dealing is frowned upon by everybody.

Alcohol has long been discouraged at the gatherings, with the hobos and winos maintaining their own "A-Camp" apart from the others. (They also pass around a "magic hat" for booze runs, but don't mistake it for the real one!) In contrast, at the European gatherings there is a tradition of moderate alcohol use as opposed to abstinence-versus-abuse polarization. This is now starting to take hold at the US gatherings, with a little discreet wine-sipping going on. There are also cannabis-free camps, just like alcohol-free and tobacco-free camps.

🍁 *Police action in the past has been heavy-handed, but more recent gatherings have passed off peacefully, with police often more bemused than concerned about arrests.*

KNOW THE LAW

As noted in the "Lows" section, the Rainbow Gathering's biggest difficulty with the authorities is a lot less to do with people smoking cannabis at the camps than the simple legal right to gather. However, there is still a need for smokers to use their common sense. The police watch the roads leading to the gatherings and use such things as a broken tail light as an excuse to stop and search a vehicle and bust people for all manner of offenses, including possession of cannabis. Within the camps, however, the security volunteers are concerned only with behavior toward other gatherers and the environment, and not what an individual might be smoking.

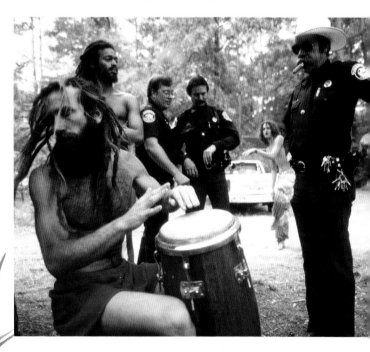

BARCELONA
SPANNABIS **SPAIN**

Barcelona, Spain's principal port and industrial hub, is its most progressive and culturally open city, too. It is also home to Spannabis—Fería del Cáñamo y Tecnologías Alternativas—the world's largest expo of hemp and cannabis-related products.

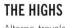

BARCELONA

Old Town

Parc de Montjuïc

Puerto

Mediterranean Sea

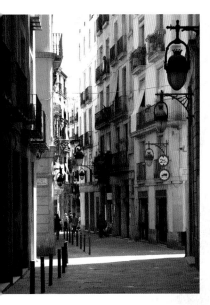

🍁 *In recent years, Barcelona's Gothic Quarter, also known as the Cathedral Quarter, has moved upmarket, but it is still home to some spectacular historic architecture.*

During the Spanish Civil War, between 1936 and 1937, Barcelona was taken over by anarchists, who collectivized the shops and factories and ran the city in open councils. Since the reestablishment of democracy after the death in 1975 of fascist dictator Francisco Franco, Barcelona has reasserted itself as the capital of Catalonia, an autonomous region within Spain with its own distinct language and culture. Helpfully for the marijuana smoker, cannabis is widespread and relatively tolerated.

THE HIGHS

Alterno-travelers might want to check into one of the hotels around the Ciutat Vella, or Old City—the medieval port. In addition to such gems as a wall near the Gothic cathedral dating to the Roman era, this area hosts a virtual carnival every night, with street musicians, fire-jugglers, fortune-tellers, and the like putting on a show for the tourists. Ciutat Vella's main drag is the scene of this spectacle—the Ramblas, which stretches from the Plaça de Catalunya on the northwest edge of the district to the waterfront.

The Ramblas bisects Ciutat Vella. On the northeast side is the Barri Gòtic, or Gothic Quarter, which has become slightly upscale, with lots of shops, bars, and cafés. On the other side are the Raval and Barri Xino—Chinatown, although today it is more Arab, East Indian, and African than Chinese. A maze of narrow streets and alleyways, this side of the Ramblas is considerably seedier, although also more flavorful. Immigrants merge with skateboarding punks and book-toting bohemians. The main artery in this section is the Rambla del Raval.

On Raval's Ramelleres Street is the headquarters of the Associació Lliure Antiprohibicionista (Free Anti-prohibitionist Association), Catalonia's foremost drug-legalization organization and a good place to check in for info on local cannabis enforcement and activist efforts to oppose it.

Barcelona has a number of world-class museums, including the Museum of Contemporary Art in Sant Antoni, the Picasso Museum on Montcada Street, and the Joan Miró Museum at Parc de Montjuïc. But the city's top tourist attraction is the Church of the Sagrada Familia, under construction since 1882, the grand vision of eccentric visionary architect Antoni Gaudí. Many of Gaudí's other creations around the city draw cannabis-enhanced tourists who grok on the wavy brickwork and flowing, earthy aesthetic that

borders on the psychedelic—particularly the Casa Milà, at 92 Passeig de Gràcia, some ten blocks from the Sagrada Familia. It's popularly known as La Pedrera, or the Quarry, for its cavelike atmosphere, said to be Gaudí's homage to the chthonic forces of the Earth. It's slightly ironic that Gaudí has become a hippie icon, as he was actually a conservative Catholic.

In the Gràcia district, the Plaça del Sol is a student and hippie convergence point with guitars strummed and bongos beaten late into the night. In August, this area hosts the Festas de Gràcia, a five-day street-arts festival that also sees nightly parties. On a hill in the Gràcia district is Park Güell, which features more Gaudí masterworks and is yet another gathering place for nighttime street partiers.

Even the seats feature Gaudí-designed and inspired mosaics in Barcelona's beautiful Park Güell.

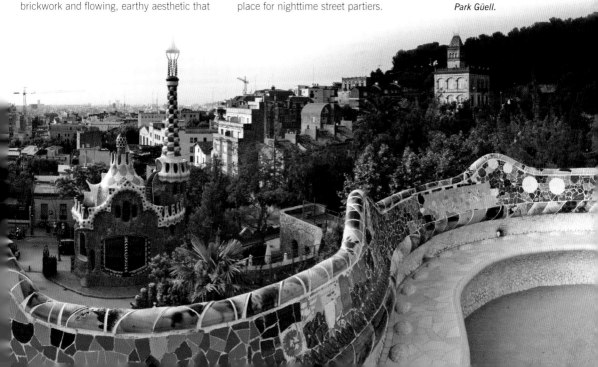

THE LOWS

Like every Mediterranean port, Barcelona has its rough areas—and the Raval/Xino district is one of them. Getting lost in the warren of alleys after dark might not be such a good idea. On the other hand, Barcelona rather too aggressively cleaned up in preparation for the 1992 Olympics, with an area of cheap, lively, music-filled bars and restaurants outside Ciutat Vella razed. This coincided with a crackdown on public cannabis use from which the city's tokers have never quite recovered. Which brings us to...

THE DOPE

Cannabis use is widespread if not entirely open around several points in the city, including the Ramblas. There is a certain amount of street peddling in Barri Xino—but also pretty heavy policing. Moroccan hashish (of varying qualities) abounds and is called *xocolát* (chocolate). Domestic Catalan homegrown is also starting to make inroads into the market, although this is more available through personal networks than street dealers. Amazingly, there is actually graffiti helpful to potential purchasers on many walls in Barcelona—black squares warn where police cameras operate and ganja leaves advertize dealing areas.

THE FESTIVAL

Since 2004, the Fira de Cornellá convention center on the city's hilly western edge has hosted Spannabis. Over 150 exhibitioners display industrial-hemp clothing and paper, growing equipment, smoking (and cleaner vaporization) paraphernalia, and samples from the world's leading cannabis seed banks.

Held for three days around late February and early March, Spannabis draws some 19,000 participants, mostly from around Europe—it is the Continent's key networking event for hemp entrepreneurs, canna-biologists, and other devotees of the plant. The 2009 Spannabis was on the theme of the

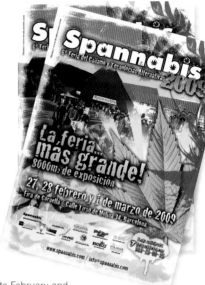

🌿 *Posters for Spannabis 2009. The exhibition is one of the largest cannabis-related events in the world.*

🌿 *A series of shots showing a bong in action. Paraphernalia of every type imaginable is found at the exhibition.*

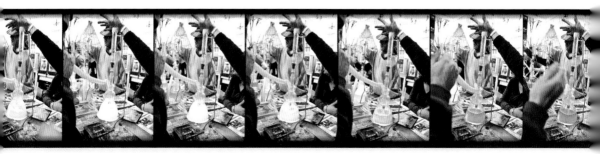

Dope Sheet

🌿 **THE PRODUCT:** Most cannabis is smoked in the form of Moroccan hash, although homegrown is becoming more popular.

🌿 **LOOK OUT FOR:** The Ramblas; a vibrant nightlife that keeps going until dawn; well-heeled shopping malls; Gaudí and other spectacular architecture, notably the Sagrada Familia and Park Güell; the Museum of Contemporary Art.

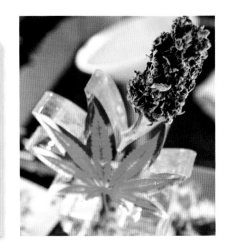

Therapeutic Qualities of Cannabis, bringing together scientists and medical doctors with cultivators, patients, and activists for seminars and workshops.

Growers also hold a Cannabis Champions Cup, second only to Amsterdam's Cannabis Cup as the world's foremost honor in the field of marijuana cultivation.

Spain plays host to another similar event, called Expocannabis, at La Cubierta convention center in Madrid, held around late October and early November.

KNOW THE LAW

Spain decriminalized cannabis in 1983, although in 1992, coinciding with the Barcelona Olympics, a law was passed instating fines for public use. There is no penalty for simple possession,

and cops in Barcelona generally warn public smokers to cut it out before actually citing them. There are criminal penalties for dealing (which can be simply passing a joint)—including prison—but with discretion left to the judge on whether the quantities involved merit severe punishment. There is no medical-marijuana law in Spain, but judges tend to take medical need into consideration. Seeds are legal and openly sold at grow-stores.

🌿 *A bud on display at Spannabis, where the Cannabis Champions Cup is awarded to the best grower.*

🌿 *Two men smoke a pipe at Spannabis 2009. The fair is an excellent place to meet people and network.*

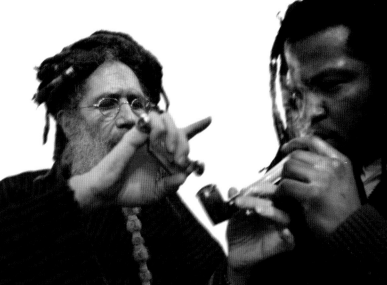

BOSTON FREEDOM RALLY USA

It is appropriate that the birthplace of the American Revolution today hosts the Northeast's biggest cannabis festival—especially given that the organizers have long been waging a free-speech struggle to keep the event alive.

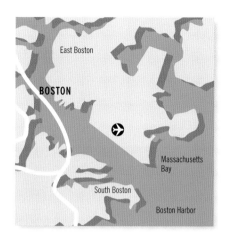

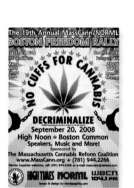

The 2008 Boston Freedom Rally poster with its decriminalization message.

Patriots and history buffs will want to walk the 2½-mile (4-kilometer) Freedom Trail that includes Boston Common, the Paul Revere house, the USS *Constitution* ("Old Ironsides"), the Old State House, and Bunker Hill.

THE HIGHS

Great eateries are to be found in Chinatown—also the city's bohemian enclave—the Italian district of North End and, across town, the Ethiopian, Japanese, Korean, and Thai establishments of South End. The nearby African American quarter of Roxbury was one of the country's hottest jazz scenes in the 1950s, and the local jazz joint Wally's Café at 427 Massachusetts Avenue, dates from this time. Also in

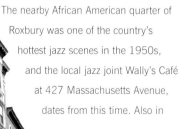

Boston's North End hosts the city's Little Italy area.

South End is Boston's anarchist bookstore and infoshop, the Lucy Parsons Center, at 549 Columbus Avenue. The more fashion-conscious will want to check out Hempest, the city's organic hemp clothing store, at 207 Newbury Street in the Back Bay East section.

THE LOWS

Despite being politically liberal, Boston has a reputation for being staid, snobbish, reserved, and generally buttoned-down. To an extent, this is an outdated cliché—the old "blue blood" elite has certainly been watered down since its heyday in the late 19th century—but the city still closes early, with the notable exception of Chinatown.

THE DOPE

New England homegrown, of variable quality, is available in the fall just as students are returning to school, and the convergence of the local outdoor harvest and the start of the fall semester floods the Boston market. The more reliably potent West Coast hydroponic and some local indoor varieties are more expensive.

THE FESTIVAL

The Massachusetts Cannabis Reform Coalition (MASS CANN))—which is the state chapter of the National Organization for the Reform of Marijuana Laws (NORML)—holds the Freedom Rally on the third Saturday of each September. The event is the East Coast's largest annual gathering to advocate marijuana-law reform.

The first rally was held in 1989 in Pittsfield; since 1995 it has been held at the Common's Carty Parade Field. The event has survived attempts by the authorities to shut it down, with suit and countersuit reaching the courts. After Hurricane Ivan washed out the 2004 rally, MASS CANN was deeply in debt, but supporters came through and the organization survived. The Freedom Rally is still going strong, drawing some 50,000.

Other than the musical talent, there are loads of vendors and political groups on hand, and speakers from national NORML and *High Times* magazine as well as MASS CANN. Unfortunately, the event usually sees some 50 to 75 arrests. The night before the festival MASS CANN holds an awards ceremony for local and national drug-policy-reform activists.

Dope Sheet

🌿 **THE PRODUCT:** Locally produced New England homegrown abounds in the fall; for a generally stronger smoke, however, look for West Coast and local hydroponic varieties.

🌿 **LOOK OUT FOR:** Walk the Freedom Trail to relive the early days of the American revolution. Restaurants to suit all tastes— head to North End for Italian, South End for eastern flavors; Chinatown; the Lucy Parsons Center for books; Hempest for organic clothing.

KNOW THE LAW

Thanks to a historic 2008 voter initiative, marijuana has been decriminalized in Massachusetts. Possession by adults of small amounts is a civil offense, subject to a fine like a traffic ticket—although possession of greater quantities and cultivation and sale can incur larger fines and/or prison sentences of varying lengths.

🌿 *The Boston Freedom Rally celebrated its 20th year in September 2009. Numerous bands and speakers entertain an audience 50,000 strong from noon till 6.00pm.*

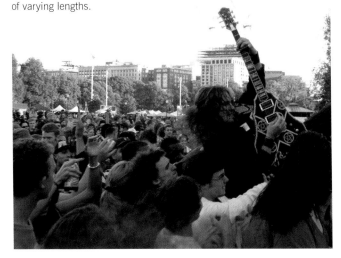

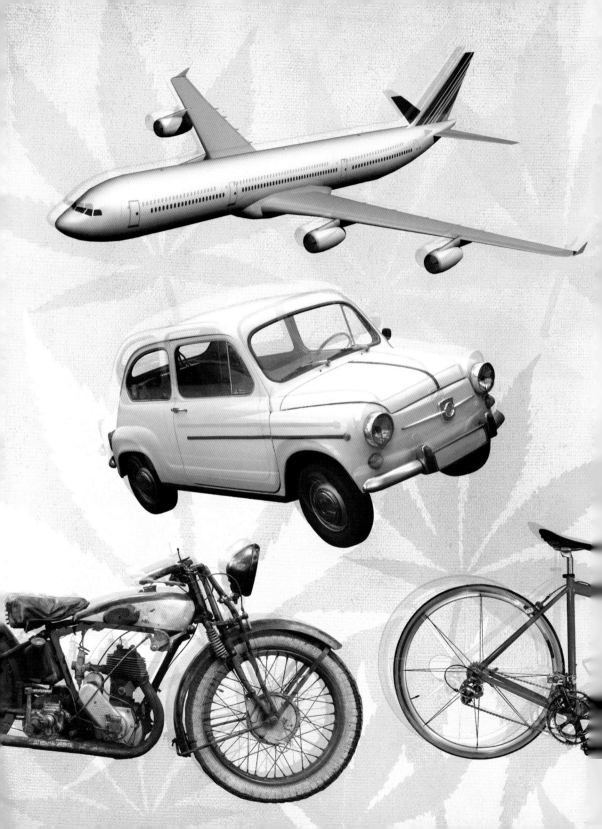

CITY TRIPS

Despite an almost global ban on the recreational use of cannabis, with discretion and a common-sense attitude you can travel the world and enjoy a smoke in some very cool places. From urbane Europe, where smoking bud will set you up for a highly cultured tour of some magnificent cities, to the chilled-out beaches of Thailand and Mexico, and the mind-expanding spirituality of India and Nepal, here's a selection of places that will have your cerebral cortexes revved up. Let's hit the road.

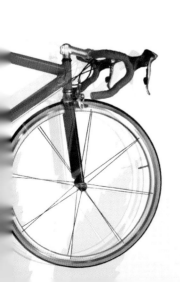
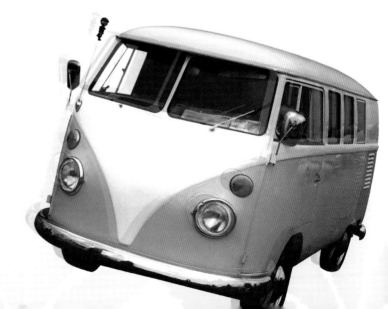

Know the Law

If, when you're traveling the world, your intention is to sample some of the cannabis that's on offer locally, it pays to know the risks you're taking—in some places you may not think they're worth it.

Although levels of tolerance for cannabis vary widely worldwide, nearly every nation on Earth is a party to the 1961 Single Convention on Narcotic Drugs, which establishes uniform "schedules" for controlled substances—with tokers' favorite herb in the most restrictive schedule. Nations have the right to establish their own enforcement policies, ostensibly in consultation with the United Nations Office on Drugs and Crime.

The USA, with the most restrictive laws in the West, led the way in the development of this system. Opiates and cocaine are Schedule 2, as drugs with legitimate medical uses; marijuana is Schedule 1, for those supposedly without. In 1970, Congress passed the Controlled Substances Act, which adopted the schedule system as US law. Currently, the USA arrests some 1.8 million people on drug charges annually, compared with just over a half million for violent crime. Around fifty percent of these are for pot violations—there have been more than twenty million marijuana arrests in the USA since 1965. Large-scale marijuana cultivators and traffickers may actually be sentenced to death under an amendment to the 1994 Violent Crime Control and Law Enforcement Act.

Not all countries conform to the Single Convention's schedules, and some have very tolerant enforcement policies—although, contrary to popular belief, cannabis is technically illegal even in the Netherlands. There, cannabis is a Schedule 2 drug and opiates are Schedule 1, in a reversal of the UN (and US) policy. Under the "Dutch model," cannabis is decriminalized, and the fines that are technically on the books for possession are not necessarily enforced.

Other European countries that have decriminalized include Spain, Italy, and Belgium—although the enforcement policy in these countries is nowhere near as liberal as in the Netherlands. Italy especially has been cracking down in recent years. In 2001, Portugal became the only European country to remove penalties for personal possession from the books entirely—which drug policy wonks consider true decriminalization as

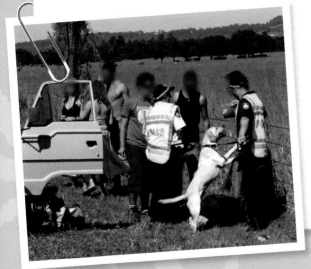

🌿 *Australian police stop and search a car on its way to Nimbin Mardi Grass.*

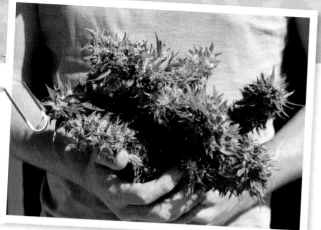

drugs. A month earlier, three former Latin American presidents—Colombia's César Gaviria, Brazil's Fernando Cardoso, and Mexico's Ernesto Zedillo—jointly released a public statement that the Washington-led drug war has failed and that decriminalization should be explored as an alternative. Issued by the Latin American Commission on Drugs and Democracy, their report states: "Prohibitionist policies based on the eradication of production and on the disruption of drug flows as well as on the criminalization of consumption have not yielded the expected results. We are farther than ever from the announced goal of eradicating drugs." There is plenty of evidence that prohibitionist strategies have backfired, and US production of marijuana now equals that of Colombia.

The information in this book only reflects the situation at the time of writing—so watch the news about your destination. No matter where you go, if you want to avoid a nasty stay in jail, execution by firing squad or public hanging, or (at best) a hefty bribe or fine—know the local law before you light up.

opposed to the "depenalization" that exists elsewhere. In Germany in 1994, the Federal Republic's top court ruled that states and localities had the option to drop criminal penalties for personal possession, and most of them have. Switzerland and the Czech Republic have both seen decriminalization bills narrowly defeated in recent years. Russia, a seemingly unlikely candidate, decriminalized personal quantities of all drugs in 2004.

In Latin America, Colombia decriminalized by a ruling of the judiciary in 1994. Venezuela passed a decrim law in 2004, and Brazil followed suit two years later. A decriminalization bill has been passed in Mexico, but not yet signed into law.

At the other end of the spectrum, China, Indonesia, the Philippines, and Malaysia have the world's most draconian enforcement policies, and you can get the death penalty for simple possession.

Dissent is emerging to the Single Convention system. In March 2009, Bolivia's President Evo Morales publicly chewed a coca leaf at the Vienna summit of the UN Commission for Narcotic Drugs to make the point that the plant should be removed from the list of prohibited

 Growing cannabis can lead to heavy fines or imprisonment.

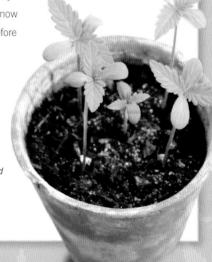

AMSTERDAM
NETHERLANDS

Amsterdam is probably the world's top cannabis destination, and with good reason, as it is one of the most wide-open cities on the planet—pulling this off without losing any of its sense of civilized European style.

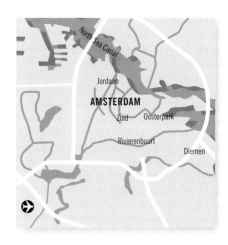

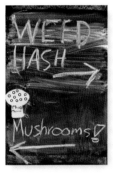

🍁 *Even in Amsterdam, a little more discretion and etiquette are expected than this.*

🍁 *Amsterdam's canals and historic buildings are popular attractions for visitors.*

As recently as two generations ago, Amsterdam was actually one of Europe's most conservative cities, but the radical youth movement of the 1960s—pioneered by the famous Provos—changed all that. The group gained notoriety with the big protest it held against the marriage of Princess Beatrix and Wehrmacht veteran Claus von Amsberg in March 1966.

The Provos campaigned against air pollution, traffic congestion, the tobacco industry—and marijuana prohibition. As Amsterdam's town fathers started adopting some of their ideas—including their White Bicycle sharing program, a prototype

that is now being adopted in a number of European cities—several Provo veterans wound up on the city council. As cannabis cultivation proliferated on Amsterdam's houseboats in the 1970s, the city's attitude toward drugs became Dutch national policy.

THE HIGHS

The famous cannabis-friendly coffeeshops are mostly located in the city's historic center—the Centrum—and the nearby red-light district. The Centrum also hosts the daily spectacle of musicians, clowns, and other

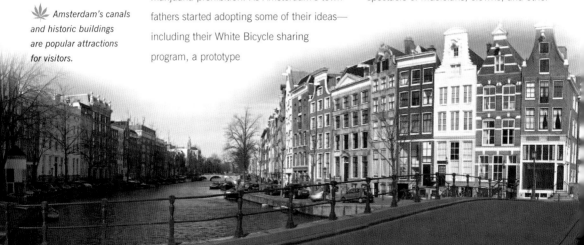

street performers (especially along the café-lined Rembrandtsplein), and it affords easy access to the city's many attractions, including the Rijksmuseum (State Museum), with its collection from the Dutch masters, the Van Gogh Museum, the Botanical Museum for those whose herbal interests extend beyond the obvious, the Heineken museum for beer enthusiasts, plus a vodka museum, a houseboat museum, a tulip museum, a sex-and-erotica museum, and a museum of Amsterdam's Jewish culture. Also located in the city center is the Anne Frank House, where you can view the original diary the girl wrote while hiding from the Nazis.

Many visitors rarely venture beyond the Centrum, where the railway station (Centraal Station) serves as a kind of hub. It's the oldest part of the city, separated by canals from newer districts. The main drags are Damrak and Rokin. To the east of the Damrak is the Old Side (Oude Zijde), marking the site of the original 13th-century settlement. Also here is the red-light district (Rossebuurt), where prostitution is officially tolerated and blatantly displayed. Also on this side is the old Jewish Quarter and the city's Chinatown. West of the Damrak is the New Side (Nieuwe Zijde)—still dating from medieval times. Walking out from the center is like journeying through time. To the south lie the 17th-century Leidseplein theater district and Canal Ring (shaped by the three city-long canals of Prinsengracht, Keizersgracht, and Herengracht). Beyond this is the 19th-century Museum Quarter.

THE LOWS

It's a contradiction that Amsterdam remains prim and conservative in unexpected ways. Even cannabis use is tightly regulated. If you insist on driving (it's easy to get around by foot, bicycle, or tram), pay close attention to all signs and signals. There is a zero-tolerance policy for all traffic violations; you can expect tickets and heavy fines even for a first offense.

The red-light district can get a little seedy after dark, despite close government regulation of the sex industry. Watch out for pickpockets. Also, be forewarned that taking photos of the

🍁 *Amsterdam has a rich architectural history, with many fine gothic, baroque, Renaissance, and Art Deco buildings.*

🍁 *Graffiti and bicycles are common in Amsterdam; the former, however, is actively discouraged—with offenders having to pay the cleaning costs.*

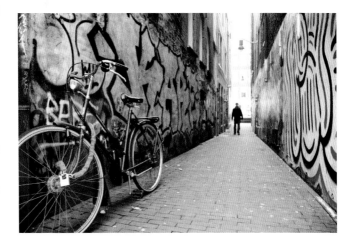

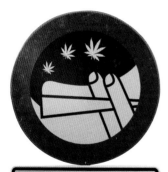

blowverbod
wegens overlast in de buurt
boete € 50,- art. 2.8 lid 2 APV

🌿 *It's illegal to smoke cannabis in outdoor areas in Amsterdam.*

🌿 *Most of the marijuana consumed in Amsterdam's coffeeshops is grown indoors.*

"window prostitutes" on display is absolutely forbidden. If you don't want a biker goon to appear out of nowhere and throw your camera into the canal, don't do it. Taking photos in the coffeeshops is also frowned upon.

A backlash threatens the city's libertine ethic. Conservative politicians have launched moves to limit the sale of cannabis to local residents as well as raising the drinking age. 2009 saw police evictions of three squatter buildings, with the riot squad mobilized and several youths arrested. The more respectful cannabis tourists are, the easier it will be for the forces of freedom to prevail against this building backlash.

THE DOPE

From locally grown indoor Nederwiet (Nether-weed) to imported Moroccan, Lebanese, and Afghani hashish, the stuff is reasonably priced in the coffeeshops. Smokers can often get a better deal for three-gram (0.1-ounce) bags, and most places supply rolling papers and filter tips. (To get an even better deal, they take a day trip to Rotterdam.) Amsterdam is a world-class cannabis-cultivation center with new hybrid strains always being developed. These are advertised openly at the coffeeshops with such alluring monikers as Double Bubble, Caramelicious, and Flying Dutchman.

Etiquette dictates that you should get something to drink as well as smoke at coffeeshops—although they generally don't serve alcohol. Keep buying drinks if you are hanging out at a table for a long time, and only smoke what you buy at that establishment.

Cannabis-laden "spacecakes" can also be had for those who prefer ingesting to inhaling—Cafe 36 in the red-light district specializes in these. Spacecakes can be really potent, so it advisable not to eat more than one at a time, and lightweights (physically or metaphorically) should just have a half. Anyone eating cannabis may be facing several hours of quasi-tripping and it is better to be safe than sorry.

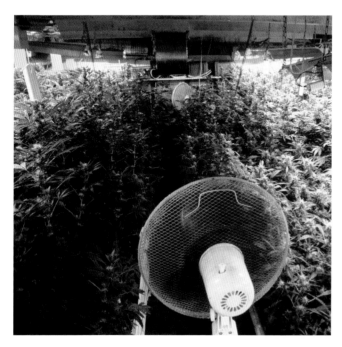

Dope Sheet

THE PRODUCT: Numerous varieties of "Nederwiet" freely available in the coffeeshops; hash from Morocco, Lebanon, and Afghanistan is also available.

LOOK OUT FOR: The Red Light district, it's not just for those "buying;" the Rijksmuseum and the Van Gogh Museum; a tour of the Heineken factory; a vibrant café and youth culture sits comfortably with more mature cultural activities.

Since an antitobacco ordinance took effect in 2008, it has been illegal to light up a cigarette in restaurants, hotels, bars, and coffeeshops in the Netherlands. This doesn't apply to cannabis, but it does put a cramp in the traditional European practice of mixing tobacco and pot in hand-rolled joints. Proprietors can set up a separate room or glass partition behind which patrons can smoke, but customers cannot be served there (to protect staff from carcinogenic fumes). Coffeeshop owners are challenging the law in the courts.

KNOW THE LAW

Drug enforcement in the Netherlands falls under the policy of "gedogen," or tolerance. Personal quantities of cannabis are freely available to anyone over the age of 18. You can buy a daily maximum of 5 grams (0.17 ounce) in the coffeeshops; 5 grams is

The original Bulldog 90 was one of the first coffeeshops in Amsterdam to sell cannabis. The Bulldog brand has now grown into a global business.

also the cut-off for what is considered personal possession, but anything under 30 grams (c. 1 ounce) is often treated with leniency. Although cultivation is ostensibly not covered by the gedogen policy (and there are signs of the authorities cracking down) it is nonetheless widespread and tolerated as long as it remains discreet. Coffeeshops are allowed to stock up to 500 grams (1.1 pounds) of cannabis— and they have to get it from somewhere.

Public smoking of cannabis is (officially, at least) not tolerated on the streets. At the moment, the situation is, paradoxically, that cannabis can only be smoked indoors and tobacco can only be smoked outdoors. The policy is actually somewhat more restrictive for tobacco!

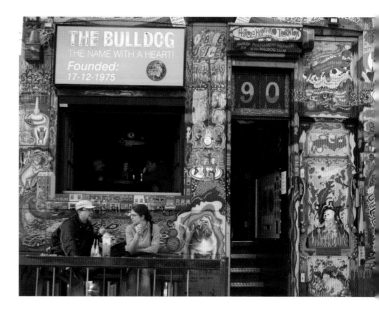

GENEVA
SWITZERLAND

Geneva's reputation as a clean and efficient center of world diplomacy and finance is certainly well earned. Beautifully situated on the shores of Lake Geneva, it is home to the world's tallest fountain, historic cathedrals, dazzling rose gardens, and the European headquarters of the United Nations.

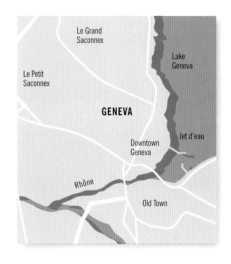

B ut alongside this slightly elitist face, Geneva is also a center for alternative culture, with a flourishing underground arts scene. There's a thriving squatter community —although this is now under attack from gentrification and a conservative backlash. This backlash has not (yet) extended to cannabis use, however. Although the weed is not officially decriminalized as it is in the Netherlands, Switzerland has a "harm reduction" policy that deemphasizes enforcement for the personal use of "soft" drugs.

THE HIGHS

The river Rhône bisects the city, with the oldest quarter on the south side. Standard tourist draws here include the birthplace of philosopher Jean-Jacques Rousseau on the Grand-Rue. The Île Rousseau, an island in Lake Geneva accessible by bridge, has a small monument to the Enlightenment thinker and is a popular spot with alternative youth. The St-Pierre Cathedral, where John Calvin preached during the Reformation, has a tower that affords breathtaking views of the city, lake, and surrounding mountains.

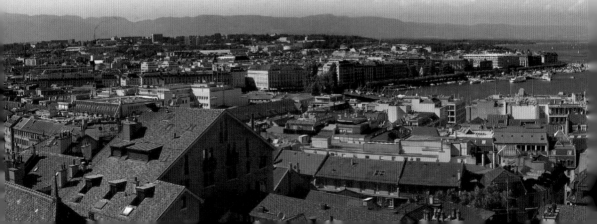

There are lots of museums—if you really want to know you're in Switzerland, check out the Horology Museum, which chronicles the history of clock and watch making in the city. Philosophy-heads will also want to visit the Voltaire Museum, home to some 24,000 editions of works about Voltaire, an avatar of intellectual freedom, and the 18th century.

For less heady nocturnal activities there are plenty of jazz and rock clubs. L'Usine, the main alternative-music venue in Geneva, is in a converted factory at Place des Volontaires 4, near the river's south shore. It features the city's hippest bands as well as the latest electronica and house music.

And there are numerous annual festivals that occasion much sophisticated European-style revelry. In June, the Fête de la Musique features scores of acts at outdoor venues spread throughout the city—featuring anything from jazz to reggae to trip-hop. In August, the Fêtes de Genève is the highlight of the summer—a ten-day party along the lakeshore with carnival rides, concerts,

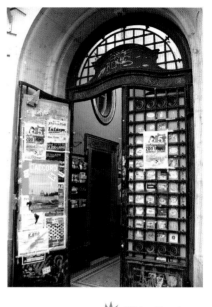

parades, and nightly fireworks. The festival culminates in a Techno Parade, with each float a rave-on-wheels, outrageously clad dancers pulsating to electro-beats. But the real event for alterno-travelers is September's La Bâtie festival where avant-garde visual and performance artists from throughout France and Switzerland stage a week of outdoor events.

Of interest to history buffs is the Fête de l'Escalade, held each December to commemorate the successful defense of the city against the 1602 invasion by the Duke of Savoy—a proud symbol of Switzerland's traditions of democracy, independence, and neutrality. The climax is a torchlight procession of over a thousand marchers dressed in period costumes through the city.

L'Usine (French for "the factory") has been Geneva's premier alternative music venue for around twenty years.

Geneva is an attractive city, located on the banks of the lake that shares its name, and nestling between two mountain chains, the Alps and the Jura.

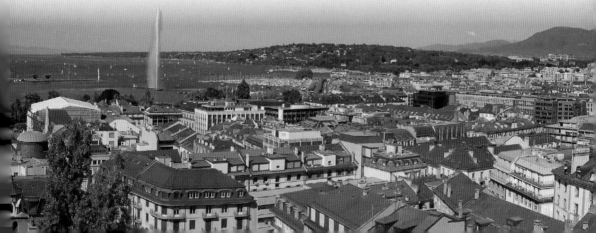

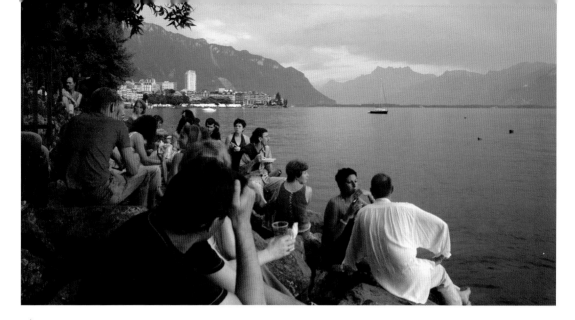

The summer months see Genevese enjoying evening drinks by the beautiful lakeside.

Northern Lights is just one of the common varieties of bud that can be found in Geneva.

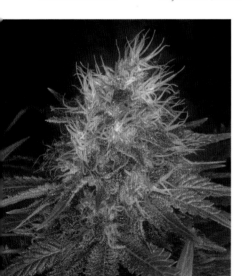

THE LOWS

Geneva's alternative culture, while still strong, is currently undergoing something of a contraction. Two of the city's premier alternative spaces have closed in recent years. The Rhino squat, which hosted the Cave Douze music collective, was evicted in July 2007. (Cave Douze continues to exist, although without a permanent space.) The following year, the Artamis cultural center, established in 1996 on an abandoned industrial site and housing hundreds of artists and musicians, was forced to close by the city fathers. There are still plenty of squats and alternative spaces, but fewer each year.

Throughout the 1980s and 1990s, there were more squats per capita in Geneva than in any other European city. Today, these are increasingly being replaced by condos. Geneva is also one of the priciest cities in Europe. So there is a sense of enjoying what could be the last gasp of one of the Continent's foremost alternative scenes before the developers take over.

THE DOPE

Swiss outdoor homegrown as well as North African hashish and the standard varieties of European greenhouse bud (Northern Lights, White Widow, etc.) are sold fairly openly at several locations around Geneva. Certain spots along the lakeshore seem to be de facto tolerance zones where those who wish to can score in relative safety. There are gatherings of people from all walks of life enjoying music, drinking wine, and having a smoke.

KNOW THE LAW

Cannabis is officially outlawed by Switzerland's 1951 Federal Narcotics Act, but the country's 26 cantons are given wide leeway in terms of enforcement and penalties. In 1991, the Swiss federal government officially adopted a "harm-reduction" policy aimed at "reducing problems related to drug use". Enforcement still varies from canton to canton, but in the urban centers police generally have adopted a reasonably lenient policy where personal quantities of cannabis are concerned—unless the user is indiscreet or obnoxious. Common-sense caution is recommended. One source warns: "The later one stays on the streets of Geneva the more likely one will be questioned by police. Being a Roma, or looking like one, might get you stopped by the police as they are quite strict with their elitist immigration policy." Attempts to decriminalize possession and consumption of cannabis have been narrowly voted down by the Federal Assembly in recent years, so there are signs of movement in the right direction.

Dope Sheet

🌿 **THE PRODUCT:** Numerous different varieties of European greenhouse bud, outdoor homegrown, and imported North African hash are available.

🌿 **LOOK OUT FOR:** The old quarter; the Horology and Voltaire museums; throughout the summer there are a number of festivals; the lakeside has some excellent restaurants and bars.

🌿 *The Artamis cultural center was home to hundreds of artists and musicians before it was shut down by the city's authorities.*

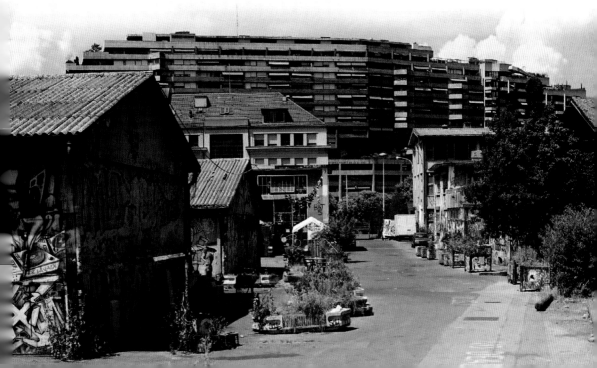

Great Cannabis Trippers of the Past

After Napoleon Bonaparte's troops discovered hashish in Egypt, the first glimmers of what would become the global cannabis culture emerged in France, with hashish becoming a muse for poets and intellectuals in the salons of Paris and Marseilles. The most celebrated personalities in this regard were Charles Baudelaire and Honoré de Balzac, both of whom were occasional patrons of the Club de Hachichins, which met in the 1840s in Paris.

Interest in this milieu was revived with the flowering of bohemian culture in the 20th century. One pioneer of this tradition was the great German-Jewish radical philosopher and cultural critic Walter Benjamin. In addition to commentaries on Baudelaire, he wrote his own memoir of the cannabis experience in 1932, *Hashish in Marseille*, which perfectly captures the apprehension of the novice user.

In the late 19th century, European adventurers had begun journeying back into the Islamic heartland of cannabis. One trailblazer was Isabelle Eberhardt, the daughter of a Swiss aristocrat who abandoned Europe for a life of adventure in North Africa. She dressed as a man, converted to Islam, and finally joined

🌿 *Isabelle Eberhardt traveled incognito in North Africa, blazing a trail for later bohemians.*

rebels fighting the colonial French. She spent the final years of her short life smoking kif in Algeria, dying in 1904 during a flash flood in the desert at the age of 27.

Eberhardt was an inspiration to the New York-born writer Paul Bowles, who translated her 1899 kif-smoking memoir *The Oblivion Seekers*. In 1931, he journeyed to North Africa himself, eventually settling in Tangier, where he wrote his best-known novel *The Sheltering Sky*. His muse as he crafted this masterpiece of travel adventure was apparently majoun, the kif-laden preparation used throughout the Maghreb. His book of short stories about life and cannabis in North Africa, *A Hundred Camels in the Courtyard*, takes its name from the Moroccan folk saying, "A pipe of kif before breakfast gives a man the strength of a hundred camels in the courtyard."

In the 1950s, a string of beatnik writers visited Bowles in Tangier, including Brion Gysin, Allen Ginsberg, Gregory Corso, Jack Kerouac, and Ira Cohen. One of these, William Burroughs, settled in Tangier himself. The city became the model for the eerie Interzone of his controversial 1959 novel *Naked Lunch*. While the book was primarily about heroin addiction (to which the author fell prey), Burroughs emphasized the distinction between heroin and cannabis, writing in his introduction: "There is no evidence that the use of any hallucinogen

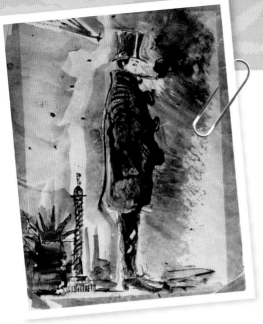

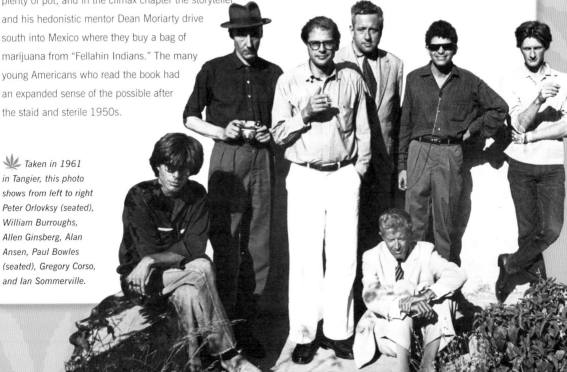

🌿 *Baudelaire's self-portrait, painted while under the influence of hashish.*

In 1960, Kerouac's real-life model for Dean Moriarty—Neal Cassady—was sprung from California's San Quentin prison after two years on a marijuana rap. He immediately sought out Ken Kesey, the young author of *One Flew Over the Cuckoo's Nest*, who was hosting LSD experiments at his home in La Honda, south of San Francisco. It was a passing of the torch from the beats to the proto-hippies.

When Kesey took his show on the road in 1965, holding "Acid Tests" up and down the coast with his band of Merry Pranksters, Cassady was the man who drove the psychedelic-painted bus. The Pranksters became the prototype for a permanent subculture of nomadic hippie adventurers that survives to this day.

results in physical dependence… A lamentable confusion between the two classes of drugs has arisen owing to the zeal of the US and other narcotic departments."

Jack Kerouac's hugely influential 1957 novel *On The Road* turned on the whole Beat Generation. There was plenty of pot, and in the climax chapter the storyteller and his hedonistic mentor Dean Moriarty drive south into Mexico where they buy a bag of marijuana from "Fellahin Indians." The many young Americans who read the book had an expanded sense of the possible after the staid and sterile 1950s.

🌿 *Taken in 1961 in Tangier, this photo shows from left to right Peter Orlovksy (seated), William Burroughs, Allen Ginsberg, Alan Ansen, Paul Bowles (seated), Gregory Corso, and Ian Sommerville.*

ESSAOUIRA
MOROCCO

Essaouira was a sleepy fishing village when the vacationing Jimi Hendrix put it on the map as a hippie destination in 1969, and Bob Marley and Cat Stevens were among the counterculture luminaries to later spend time there.

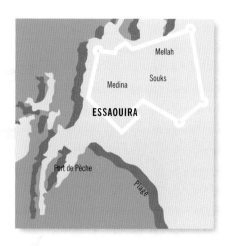

Essaouira, set on the Atlantic coastline, is a focal point for artists from all over the world, and has recently become a popular destination for kite- and wind-surfers.

It was also in 1969 that the Living Theater troupe settled in Essaouira to prepare for a tour. These 1960s adventurers likely became aware of the town as the location of Orson Welles's classic 1952 version of *Othello*. By the 1990s, tourism had surpassed fishing as the local economic pillar, but it remains comparatively low-key and alternative tourism. With lots of these types passing through, there are always hip parties going on—in a region steeped in a history of Berber rebels, sufi mystics, pirates, and kif smoking.

THE HIGHS

Essaouira has gone by a few names, reflecting its complicated history. It is known to the locals as Souira, and old maps may still show it as Mogador. A short-lived Portuguese fort, the Castelo Real de Mogador, was overrun by local warriors in 1510. Portuguese pirates continued to use the cove as a base until Sultan Muhammad bin Abd Allah established a military outpost there in 1760. These battlements are today a UN-recognized World Heritage Site.

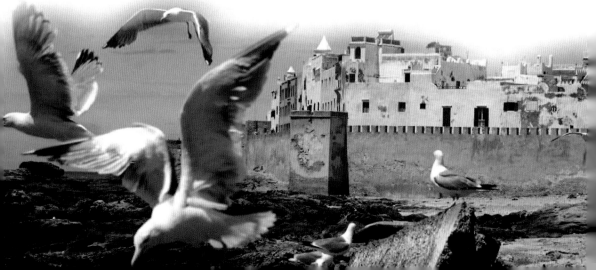

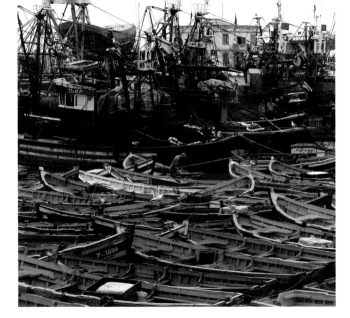

A lure for music-lovers is the local Gnawa culture. The Gnawa are both an ethnic group and a kind of religious order, whose ceremonies are centered on trance-inducing music. The Gnawa are thought to be descended from Black African slaves who were brought to Morocco after the conquest of the Songhai Empire in 1591. Today, they are a respected musical caste, putting the Arabic words of Islamic hymns to tunes and rhythms brought from sub-Saharan Africa. Essaouira hosts an annual four-day Gnawa festival that draws 450,000 people.

The town lies at a cultural crossroads, where Morocco's dominant Arab culture meets the Bedouin culture of the south and that of the Berbers in the interior mountains and desert. There are plenty of beautiful spots down the coast. Taghazoute, between Essaouira and Agadir, is Morocco's board-surfing capital, with legendary waves and

Essaouira is an important center for sufism, and pilgrims still come to the town to honor the shrines of sufi saints each spring. The town is also a site of Jewish pilgrimage, with thousands of Jews from abroad coming each September to visit the tomb of the revered 19th-century rabbi Haim Pinto. Essaouira had a thriving Jewish community before the establishment of Israel, but virtually all that is left of it today are two cemeteries. The pilgrims are still welcomed back, though.

The bustling harbor provides local fish restaurants with excellent fresh catches daily.

Gnawa people dance in the streets of Essaouira before the opening of the 10th Gnaoua World Music Festival. The event is held in June each year.

Morocco was made a French protectorate in 1912 but became independent again in 1956. This was just in time for the arrival of the beats and later the hippies. Essaouira's Damgaard Gallery, opened in the 1960s by Danish enthusiasts of Moroccan folk art, was an early outpost of hippiedom.

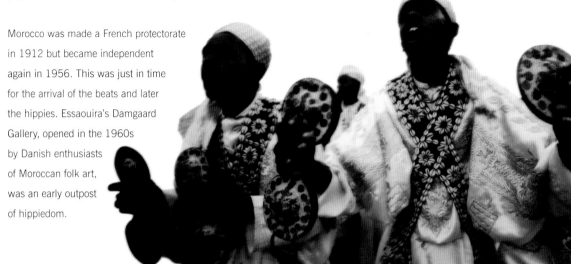

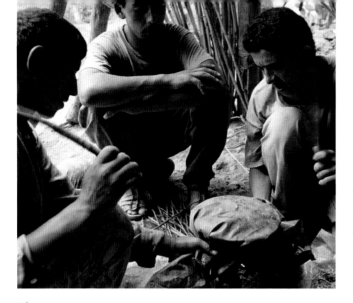

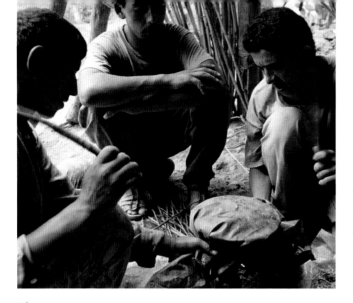 *Young farmers making hashish from marijuana leaves in the Rif Mountains, Morocco.*

tourism and economic desperation inevitably leads to the phenomenon of tourist parasitism. Lots of young men will offer to be your guide for a little compensation. Some are totally legitimate; some are scam artists who will want to take you for more than originally offered and can be hard to get rid of. Some sell marijuana, the price and quality of which will depend on what they think the buyer is worth and what they can get away with.

a laid-back party scene. Be aware that if you cross into what the government calls the Southern Provinces, you will be in what the local Bedouin consider to be Western Sahara, territory seized by Morocco when the colonial administrators of what had been Spanish Sahara withdrew in 1975. No government recognizes Morocco's claim to the territory. A ceasefire with the Polisario Front rebels has been in place since 1990, but there are periodic popular uprisings. If you go down there, be advised you are on contested land.

Accommodations in Essaouira are basic (usually no hot water), but cheap compared with points north in Morocco (already a good deal cheaper than Europe). There is great seafood, of course, and lots of pleasant waterfront restaurants.

THE LOWS

There is some pretty harsh poverty in Essaouira and its environs. The mixture of

THE DOPE

Cannabis in Morocco is generally in the form of hashish or kif—the fine powder of THC crystals shaken from the buds. (Hashish is basically kif concentrated and solidified with pressure, heating, and sometimes a solvent or binding agent—originally sweat from the hands of the hashish makers, although today more often ethanol.) Kif and hashish are widely produced in the northern Rif Mountains, and production has also moved into the interior Atlas Mountains—despite periodic spasms of eradicationist zeal on the part of the authorities.

This hashish gets all around both Europe and Morocco but is cheaper and tends to be purer in Morocco—although quality will vary, and there is still some adulterated stuff. Kif is not going to be adulterated, and because it can't be transported in easy-to-smuggle blocks, it doesn't get out of Morocco much. This is the truly unique North African experience.

The stuff is smoked in a thin long-stemmed pipe called a *sipsi*—for the clarinet-like woodwind instrument that it resembles. These are used to smoke tobacco as well as hash and kif, sometimes in combination.

One distinct local delicacy is *majoun*—an edible paste made from kif and honey with flavorings such as chopped dates, raisins, nuts, ginger, anise, and so on. This can be pretty strong, so caution is recommended by those in the know.

Travelers may be tempted to go into the hashish heartland of the Rif, but be forewarned that the cannabis-producing tribesmen are understandably paranoid about strangers. This is dangerous turf for outsiders.

Dope Sheet

THE PRODUCT: Cannabis is usually in the form of hash or kif, rarely bud. Majoun is a locally produced edible paste, made from kif—it can be extremely strong.

LOOK OUT FOR: Very unspoilt, despite growth in tourism; the area still retains a laid-back feel; cheap but good fish restaurants; the town is popular with artists, and galleries are numerous; the four-day Gnaoua World Music Festival held each June attracts 450,000 people.

KNOW THE LAW

Cannabis is illegal in the Kingdom of Morocco, and the penalty for possession is ten years in prison. Tourists have been known to be let off with only a fine or warning, but such leniency cannot be counted on—travelers should be very careful. Despite the law, Morocco does need tourist dollars, as well as the annual $7 billion that makes hashish the country's largest source of foreign currency. It is still a leading producer despite the government's claims of slashing output.

The vast majority of Moroccan marijuana is turned into hash and exported to Europe.

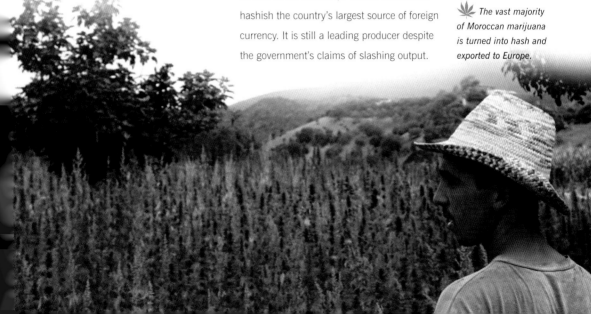

DURBAN
SOUTH AFRICA

Durban, on South Africa's Indian Ocean coast and one of the biggest ports on the continent, is synonymous among global stoners with the ultrapotent variety of *dagga* (cannabis) somewhat hyperbolically dubbed "Durban Poison."

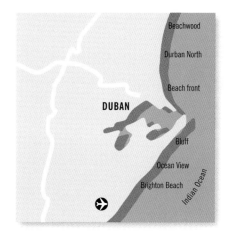

T his, along with great beaches, world-class surfing, and a year-round temperate climate, makes it an inevitable destination for herbal adventurers. KwaZulu-Natal, of which Durban is the largest city, is known as South Africa's "Garden Province," an agricultural heartland with a burgeoning wine industry. Inland, the coastal plain rises rapidly to a high plateau that stretches west to the remote and impressive Drakensberg Mountains that form the border with the Kingdom of Lesotho.

A surfer passes three swimmers taking a break at Durban Beach. During the apartheid years, this beach was segregated for whites only.

THE HIGHS

In the apartheid era, the province was called Natal, and KwaZulu was a "bantustan"—one of the ten pseudo-autonomous "homelands" the apartheid regime drew up for South Africa's black majority. KwaZulu was the bantustan for the Zulu people, and it was a noncontiguous patchwork of the poorest lands. With the end of apartheid in 1994, KwaZulu was integrated into the new province of KwaZulu-Natal.

This region was the seat of the Zulu nation and then of a Boer republic between 1839 and its annexation by Britain in 1843. Then the Boers (Dutch-speaking settlers) tried to reclaim it in the 1899 Boer War. Each of

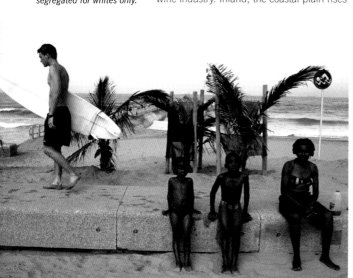

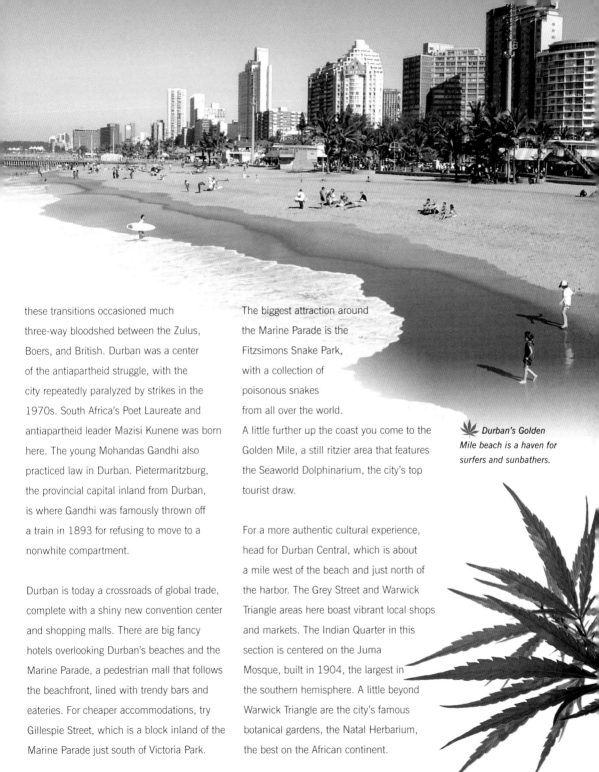

these transitions occasioned much three-way bloodshed between the Zulus, Boers, and British. Durban was a center of the antiapartheid struggle, with the city repeatedly paralyzed by strikes in the 1970s. South Africa's Poet Laureate and antiapartheid leader Mazisi Kunene was born here. The young Mohandas Gandhi also practiced law in Durban. Pietermaritzburg, the provincial capital inland from Durban, is where Gandhi was famously thrown off a train in 1893 for refusing to move to a nonwhite compartment.

Durban is today a crossroads of global trade, complete with a shiny new convention center and shopping malls. There are big fancy hotels overlooking Durban's beaches and the Marine Parade, a pedestrian mall that follows the beachfront, lined with trendy bars and eateries. For cheaper accommodations, try Gillespie Street, which is a block inland of the Marine Parade just south of Victoria Park.

The biggest attraction around the Marine Parade is the Fitzsimons Snake Park, with a collection of poisonous snakes from all over the world. A little further up the coast you come to the Golden Mile, a still ritzier area that features the Seaworld Dolphinarium, the city's top tourist draw.

For a more authentic cultural experience, head for Durban Central, which is about a mile west of the beach and just north of the harbor. The Grey Street and Warwick Triangle areas here boast vibrant local shops and markets. The Indian Quarter in this section is centered on the Juma Mosque, built in 1904, the largest in the southern hemisphere. A little beyond Warwick Triangle are the city's famous botanical gardens, the Natal Herbarium, the best on the African continent.

Durban's Golden Mile beach is a haven for surfers and sunbathers.

To connect with the city's alternative scene, seek out the Bartel Arts Trust Centre (BAT), a converted warehouse on the harbor front just off the Victoria Embankment. With its murals, and workshops in music, visual arts, dance, crafts, and literature, the BAT Centre features galleries and nightly performances by hot local bands.

For surfing, try North Beach, New Pier, Cave Rock, Dairy Beach, or Baggies. For an uncrowded and scenic beach, head for the Umhlanga Rocks, some 12 miles (20 kilometers) up the coast from Durban. Reachable by bus from Durban Central, Umhlanga has long been a reliable hippie hang-out—although quiet beachfronts are getting harder to find even there, because of tourism development. (On beaches without a shark net, be careful in the water—man-eating great whites abound.)

South of Durban is the Hibiscus Coast, stretching from Hibberdene to Port Edward. Starting about 60 miles (100 kilometers) below Durban, this refuge of sheltered coves, nature preserves, and pristine beaches provides

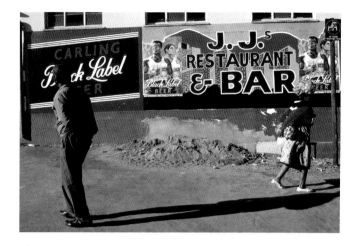

Despite the thriving tourist trade, many parts of Durban are still ravaged by poverty.

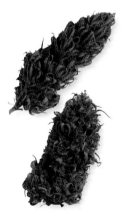

Because of the city's large port, roads around Durban are good.

an escape from the crowds if you go there off-season—meaning, not around Christmas. Below the Hibiscus Coast, across the line in eastern Cape Province and Transkei region, the homeland of the Xhosa people, is the Wild Coast—still more remote and rugged, and a well-known center of cannabis cultivation. The Wild Coast begins around Port St Johns, some 120 miles (200 kilometers) down from Durban. The Wild Coast town of Umtata (also rendered Mthatha) features a Nelson Mandela Museum. South Africa's national hero was born in the nearby village of Mvezo.

THE LOWS

Violent crime has been one of post-apartheid South Africa's biggest challenges, and Durban is no exception. Walking around

Durban Central late at night might not be the wisest move, and keep your wits about you after dark. (It's a lot safer in the more upscale Durban Beach area.) On the other side of the coin, runaway tourism development is eating into space for authentic culture—the usual dilemma. The rural areas are less dangerous.

THE DOPE

Like skunkweed in Northern California, Durban Poison (DP) is a sort of Holy Grail for aficionados—a legendary high-potency strain which has largely been lost to hybridizing. But, while skunk is an indica-heavy hybrid, DP is almost pure sativa—therefore producing a very "up," cerebral high, perfect for hiking along a deserted beach, checking out the scenery. Lots of internet seed emporiums claim to sell DP, but it is doubtful if this is always the stuff that became legendary in the 1970s. The original DP came wrapped around a stick, like the Thai stick that was widely available in the USA in the same era. Post-DP varieties can sometimes still be had in this form, known as "fingers," at reasonable rates. Shorter sticks are called Pietermaritzburg Slugs.

Other varieties available are Swazi Red and Malawi Gold—imported from, respectively, Swaziland and Malawi, of course. Cannabis is known locally as *dagga* and is commonly sold on the streets of Durban Central in small plastic bags, known as "bankies." A joint is a

"zol," and papers are "blades." Low-grade stuff—ubiquitous among the Central street dealers—is called "majat."

KNOW THE LAW

While the smoking atmosphere in Durban is relatively relaxed, cannabis possession is a criminal offense in South Africa. The maximum sentence for even a small quantity is 15 years, but this is rarely imposed. For tourists, a small fine is more likely. However, this is entirely at the judge's discretion, so it's perhaps best not to tempt fate. Smoking on the street or Durban Beach is not advised; smoking on more remote and quiet beaches might be OK if a reasonable degree of caution is exercised.

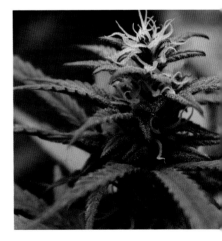

🌿 *A bud of the now legendary Durban Poison, a high-potency, sativa-rich strain.*

VARANASI
INDIA

Varanasi has perhaps the oldest and strongest local cannabis culture on the planet. Rising on the banks of the Ganges, it is India's holiest city, and its special deity is Shiva the Destroyer, the god most closely associated with cannabis.

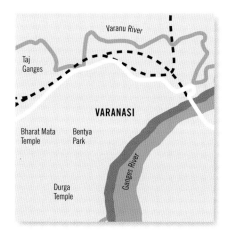

W hile the masses partake widely in *bhang*—the special cannabis preparation—at certain Hindu holy festivals, the city has a permanent population of *sadhus*, the itinerant class of spiritual seekers who have dropped out of the caste system and its rigid program of life stations in the quest for enlightenment. Described by one traveler as "thousand-year-old hippies," the sadhus can always be found imbibing and meditating on the city's *ghats*, or stone steps leading to the riverbank, usually dedicated to a Hindu deity. Since the 1960s, Varanasi's sadhus have merged with hippies and seekers from the West in an informal transient community more or less perpetually clouded in fragrant smoke.

THE HIGHS

India's drug laws don't have much chance of wiping out a 4,000-year tradition of cannabis use in the country. As far back as 2000 BCE, the Atharva Veda noted cannabis as among the "kingdoms of herbs which release us from anxiety."

Even the British colonial administration— busy as it was purchasing opium from the Indians and selling it to the Chinese—made little effort to suppress cannabis. In 1893, the Indian Hemp Drugs Commission, called

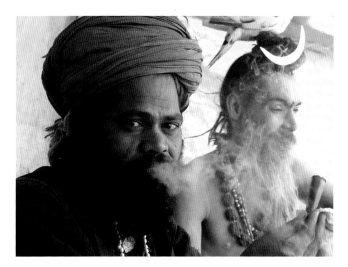

A sadhu smoking a chillum in Varanasi – 'Land of Shiva'. Smoking cannabis is rare for most of the local inhabitants, who generally only imbibe bhang during religious festivals, notably Holi.

by British colonial authorities to study the cannabis "problem" in India, warned against prohibition of bhang, and the report made special note of Varanasi's traditions. In an appendix on religious use of hemp, British bureaucrat J.M. Campbell noted references to use of bhang in the *Kashi Khanda*, the ancient sacred text about the spiritual practices in the city. (See the box below.)

J.M. Campbell on bhang

"The students of the scriptures at Benares [Varanasi] are given bhang before they sit to study. At Benares, Ujjain, and other holy places yogis, bairagis and sanyasis take deep draughts of bhang that they may Centre their thoughts on the Eternal…bhang is… victorious over the demons of hunger and thirst. By the help of bhang ascetics pass days without food or drink. The supporting power of bhang has brought many a Hindu family safe through the miseries of famine. To forbid or even seriously to restrict the use of so holy and gracious a herb as the hemp would cause widespread suffering and annoyance and to the large bands of worshipped ascetics deep-seated anger. It would rob the people of a solace in discomfort, of a cure in sickness, of a guardian whose gracious protection saves them from the attacks of evil influences."

When it is for *puja* (sacrament), bhang remains de facto legal in Varanasi as in some other Indian holy cities. During Shivaratri, the festival honoring Shiva, it is practically a duty for devotees of the god of destruction and regeneration to partake of bhang. Bhang lassis (see page 79) also flow freely at Holi, the spring festival. The national government is wise enough not to try to suppress millennia of cultural tradition, and the Uttar Pradesh state government actually registers a few small shops where the stuff is sold with official authorization.

Varanasi vies with Damascus for the title of the oldest continuously inhabited city on Earth, and cannabis use has been there from the beginning. By Hindu tradition those who die in the city achieve liberation from the cycle of death and rebirth; hence many aged pilgrims come to the city for their final days.

Varanasi is situated on the west bank of the Ganges and is one of the oldest inhabited cities in the world.

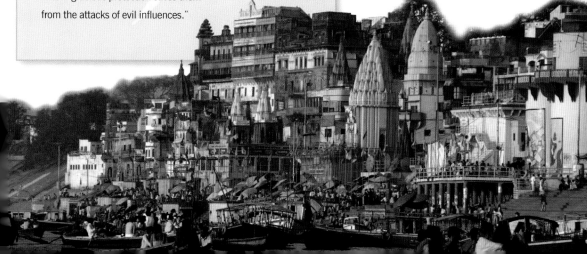

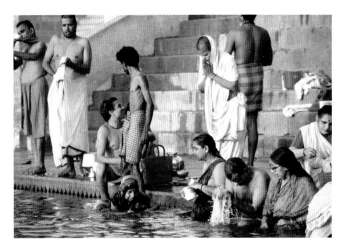

🌿 *The Ganges plays a hugely significant role in the religious lives of Hindus, as well as being a place to wash.*

🌿 *There are up to five million sadhus in India. They are noted for their spirituality and strict ascetism.*

In the 19th century, Annie Besant chose Varanasi for the Indian headquarters of her Theosophical Society, which was instrumental in reviving the high tradition of Hindu mysticism (then in decline as a result of colonial rule) and passing it on to the West—a vital precursor of the hippie and New Age movements. All these legacies are alive and well in contemporary Varanasi.

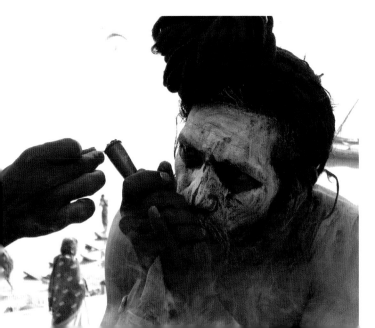

THE LOWS

Varanasi, like most Indian cities, is extremely crowded, very hot, utterly chaotic, and quite dirty. The poor bathe and drink in the Ganges because they have to, but if you're of a fragile constitution you might want to avoid even getting near it; the sacred river is quite literally full of shit, both human and animal. Homeless and sadhus alike squat where they can; so do cows and water buffalo. Endless varieties of debris flow along the river, including dead animals and attendant vultures. If you are squeamish about this sort of thing, maybe you should consider Amsterdam instead.

Like just about everywhere else in the world, Varanasi has tightened up somewhat since the high tide of hippiedom. Although an exception is made for sacramental use, India does have drug laws that conform to the international standard of the Single Convention. The sadhus may be seen as occupying a gray area between sacramental and recreational use; foreign hippies who hang with them are far less likely to be seen the same way, no matter how serious their spiritual quest, and should remain discreet.

There is much harsh poverty and human suffering in Varanasi—and, recently, a few horrific instances of terrorism, including deadly blasts at an ancient Hindu temple in 2006 and a courthouse in 2007. The good news is that if these bombings were intended to spark Hindu–Muslim communal violence in Varanasi—of the kind seen in too many parts of India in recent years—they failed. The city remained calm after both, a testament to the survival of its universalist spirit despite the onslaught of both Islamic and Hindu fundamentalism.

THE DOPE

The respectable way to consume cannabis in Varanasi is as bhang—dried buds crushed to a powder with mortar and pestle, gently roasted, and then ingested. The poor may mix their bhang with water, but the preferred way is with dairy. Most common is to mix it

Dope Sheet

🌿 **THE PRODUCT:** The normal practice is to imbibe locally produced bhang (crushed, roasted bud) mixed into lassi (a yogurt drink). Sadhus and some Westerners will smoke bud in a chillum.

🌿 **LOOK OUT FOR:** One of the world's oldest inhabited cities; an important religious center—temples exist on most street corners; Banarasi silkware and brassware, jewelry, woodcrafts, carpets; Assi Ghat is where young foreigners congregate.

🌿 *For those who can afford it, bhang is commonly mixed with lassi, a yogurt-like drink.*

with lassi, the yogurt drink that is popular throughout north India. Lassi can be either salty or sweet, and flavored with almonds, pistachios, cardamoms, peppercorns, cinnamon stick, and bhang—in any combination. The THC bonds with the milk fat, making it a more efficient means of delivery than water.

Smoking the stuff as ganja or hashish as opposed to ingesting it as bhang carries at least a slight social stigma and is left to the sadhus and foreigners.

KNOW THE LAW

The penalty for possession of personal quantities of cannabis in India is a prison sentence and/or a fine. Varanasi is the principal city where government-authorized bhang shops sell the stuff legally for use in religious ceremonies.

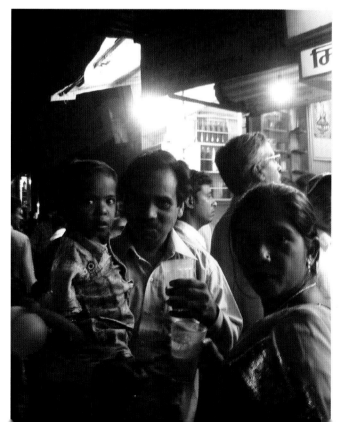

KATHMANDU
NEPAL

Despite being a world tourism destination, Kathmandu remains steeped in a centuries-old local cosmology and unique culture where the Indo-Aryan sphere of the Indian subcontinent meets the Sino-Tibetan realms of the Himalayas and China.

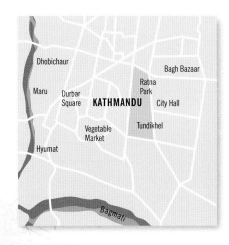

N epal's ancient tradition of hashish has made it a key cannabis-tourism destination since the 1960s—just about ten years after the Himalayan kingdom emerged from near-total isolation. Chaotic traffic and cyber-cafés coexist with ancient temples and royal palaces, and a day's travel into the mountains can seem like entering a different age.

Kathmandu provides a unique mix of ancient and modern, and is used as a base for many backpackers trekking in the foothills of the Himalayas.

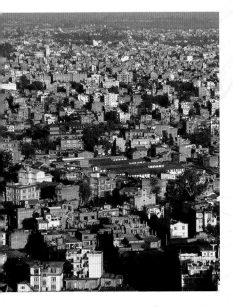

Nepal follows the Himalayas from northwest to southeast, and its distinct bioregions form belts along this same axis. In the south is the Terai, Nepal's small strip of the Ganges plain, flat and fertile. To the north of this rise the Chure and Mahabharat ranges, the first foothills of the Himalayas. Then come the Pahar midlands, which cover most of the country and include the Kathmandu Valley. Beyond this are the Himalayas proper, which rise precipitously to Mt Everest and the border with Tibet.

THE HIGHS

Kathmandu is the traditional homebase for backpacking excursions around the country, but the city is also one of the most fascinating on Earth and needs at least ten days to really do it justice. The center of old Kathmandu is Durbar Square—a UN World Heritage Site, home to palaces and several magnificent Hindu and Buddhist temples.

The main drag of upscale Kathmandu is the Durbar Marg, a broad 19th-century thoroughfare lined with expensive hotels. But to experience the magic of old Kathmandu, follow the Makhan Tole from the northeast corner of Durbar Square.

This narrow shopping street spills into Indra Chowk, the city's old thoroughfare. It passes Akash Bhairab Temple, honoring Shiva as a manifestation of the sky god, guarded by brooding lions cast in metal, and continues to the artificial lake Rani Pokhari, or Queen's Bath—created in the 17th century, with water from 51 sacred sources across Nepal. A small island in the lake contains a temple, rebuilt after a storm in 1924, to Shiva.

Hippie tourists will also want to head for Jochne Street—today known practically universally as "Freak Street," a legacy of the 1960s and 1970s when it was the local haven for counterculture vagabonds. It still is, to an extent, with plenty of cheap hotels and funky little curry shops and street stalls. This extends south from Basantapur Square—another splendid plaza bounded by ancient temples and palaces a little north and west of Durbar.

Dope Sheet

THE PRODUCT: "Temple balls" (balls of hash) are very powerful; perhaps less potent but still good are hash "fingers"; bhang lassi is also readily available.

LOOK OUT FOR: Durbar Square for palaces and temples; bustling backstreets and colorful markets, all steeped in a rich cultural heritage; head to Thamel quarter for the new hippie scene; "Freak Street" for a taste of the old hippie trail of the 1960s and 1970s.

But the new hippie scene is now in the Thamel district. To get there, continue north from the Rani Pokhari and make a left at the Garden of Dreams. This district is traditionally inhabited by the Newars, said to be the indigenous people of the Kathmandu Valley. It is today the permanent freak fest that Freak Street was 30 years ago.

Pashupatinath is the biggest and oldest Hindu temple in Kathmandu. Services in celebration of Lord Shiva are conducted by Brahmin priests from southern India.

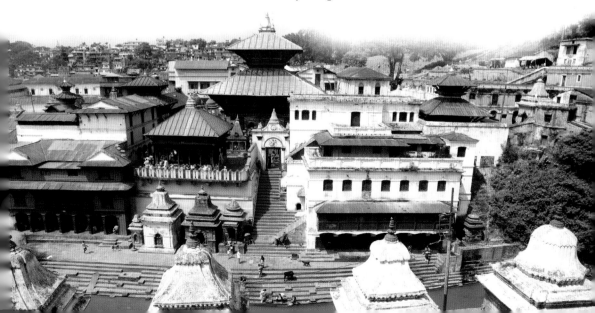

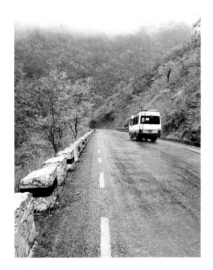

Roads in Nepal, although occasionally treacherous, will take you through some of the most spectacular scenery in the world.

THE LOWS

After years of conflict and despite the relative peace since 2006 (see the box opposite), Nepal is still a divided country. Following the proliferation of guerillas and army-backed paramilitary groups during the civil war, lots of the countryside remains contested turf where the rule of law is dubious at best. The UN recently warned of an "alarming" rise in ransom kidnappings in Nepal. Kathmandu is fairly safe, but if you decide to trek in remote areas (which are, of course, breathtakingly beautiful), it is best to have a trusted guide.

THE DOPE

As in India, sadhus and devotees of Shiva have used hashish ceremonially for centuries. It is still widely used at the spring Holi festival, when the authorities tend to turn a blind eye. However, during the rest of the year, a certain degree of caution is necessary.

Traditional hashish "temple balls"—incredibly oily, fragrant, and potent—are still available, although no longer in the temples, many of which are off-limits to non-Hindus in any case. Although illegal, hash-making remains a proud and time-honored industry. Authentic temple balls come stamped with the producer's insignia and wrapped in custom-made paper adorned with such slogans as "Blows the mind, cools the head." "Fingers" of high-quality hash are also available. There is no point in being circumspect about the fact that hash is sold openly in the Thamel area—the authorities must already know. Bhang lassi (the cannabis-spiked yogurt drink) is also pretty freely available. A lot of seemingly "legitimate" sweet shops offer this delicacy.

The Terai lowlands in the south are the prime cannabis-production area—if the least scenic part of the country—and Terai's product is available all over both Nepal and India.

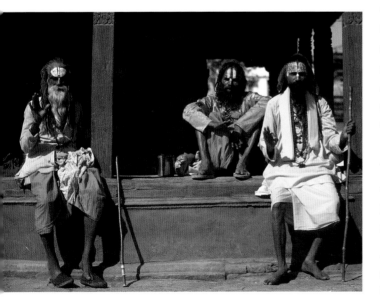

Sadhus are a common sight in Kathmandu, and are most often seen around the city's numerous temples.

KNOW THE LAW

Cannabis was outlawed in Nepal as late as 1973, when the country brought its legal code into line with the Single Convention. The very next day, the 19th-century Singha Durbar Palace that housed the parliament was destroyed by fire—probably in protest at the cannabis ban. It has since been rebuilt.

Under Nepal's Narcotics Drug Control Act, cannabis possession can be punishable by a long stretch in prison. It seems there is some reluctance to enforce this; even more rarely for tourists. However, never be complacent— tokers would be wise to keep their smoking confined to the hotel room or very secluded areas outside crowded Kathmandu.

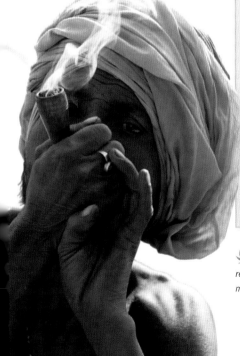

🍁 *Openly smoking in public is not recommended. It's acceptable for the many sadhus, but risky for travelers.*

Nepal between War and Peace

🍁 Nepal has had a turbulent road towards modernity, and travelers should have some savvy about the internal politics. These have been quite violent in recent years, although there is a sense that the country is back from the brink.

🍁 After a brief experiment with multi-party democracy, in 1962 King Mahendra imposed a *panchayat* system, in which localities elected councils and representatives from among traditional village elders—virtually ensuring loyalty to the throne. Protests in 1980 and 1990 finally resulted in a party-based system. But continued oppressive poverty in the countryside led to the emergence of a powerful Maoist guerilla insurgency in the late 1990s. King Birendra was killed in a palace massacre in 2001, and his brother Gyanendra assumed the throne. He dismissed the elected government in 2002 and finally took dictatorial control in February 2005. But this precipitated an alliance between the guerillas and the democratic opposition in the cities. Under a 2006 peace deal, the Maoists agreed to lay down arms in exchange for their right to stand in free elections. The monarchy was abolished in 2008, and Maoist leader Pushpa Kamal Dahal (Prachanda) was elected prime minister. However, in 2009, Prachanda's government collapsed and a coalition of rival parties took power.

🍁 So while Nepal is officially at peace, there are several intersecting undercurrents of social and political unrest that travelers should be aware of.

KOH TAO
THAILAND

Given its unforgiving drug laws, Thailand is an unlikely cannabis destination. But the Gulf of Thailand islands—justly billed as a tropical paradise—include the small jewel of Koh Tao, which is a haven for alternative travelers.

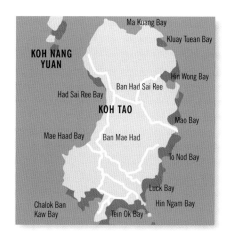

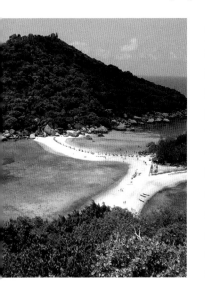

The Thai island of Koh Tao is many travelers' idea of tropical paradise. Originally uninhabited, the first residents were political prisoners who were sent to the island in 1933.

Koh Tao is Thai for "turtle island," and it is named for the sea turtles that swim and forage off the coast. Jungle cloaks the interior, palm trees line the beaches, and the snorkeling and scuba-diving off the shore are magnificent. It's a fairly open secret that a good deal of discreet smoking of very high-quality ganja goes on.

THE HIGHS

Ben Dronkers of the Netherlands Sensi Seed Bank and Cannabis Castle has established a Sensi Paradise Beach Resort on Koh Tao. It is a comfortable if slightly rustic affair (stilts, thatched roof— but also fax and Internet). One review of the establishment recommends discretion when smoking, but adds that "staff take an easy-going attitude toward the way people enjoy their holidays."

Sensi Paradise is located at the south end of Mae Haad beach on the island's west side, which is the main disembarkation point—all travel to Koh Tao is by boat, mostly from Koh Samui, which has the region's only airport. This is actually more secluded than the main populated area of Sairee Village, a ten-minute walk up the coast, lined with hotels, bars, restaurants, dive centers, cyber-cafés, and the like. Tourist highlights include a Fishery Museum and a cluster of rocks called Suan Hin Jor Por Ror with a carved inscription from King Rama V's visit in 1899. On the southern coast is Chalok Baan Kao beach, facing the islands of Koh Phangan and Koh Samui, and offering a similar range of accommodation, eateries, and nightlife. On Koh Tao, as well as better-known Phuket, full-moon parties are all the rage.

Between Koh Tao and Koh Samui is Ang Thong Marine Park, an archipelago of small

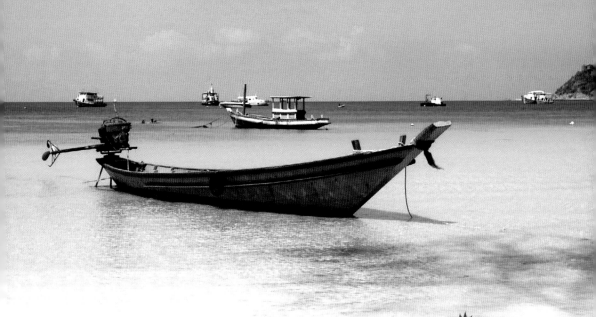

islands teeming with monkeys, birds, and other wildlife. Tours of the park can be organized from Koh Tao, although access is limited to small groups.

Even the least ambitious beach bum should really make an effort to escape the lures of Koh Tao and get around Thailand a little. The historic city of Ayutthaya—Thailand's former capital, about an hour north of Bangkok—is a UN World Heritage Site, with towering prang (reliquary towers) and gigantic monasteries.

Highs in Bangkok include the Wat Phra Keaw, or Temple of the Emerald Buddha— famous for its golden spires and green-jade Buddha. It is adjacent to the royal Grand Palace. Both were built in 1782 when Bangkok was founded. The architecturally distinctive Grand Palace looks like a European palace of that era but is crowned with traditional Thai gold-plated cupolas. Don't miss the Damnoen Saduak, or Floating Market, where an abundance of fresh fruits and vegetables are sold from small rowboats.

Wat Pho (also called Wat Phra Chetuphon) features the world's largest reclining Buddha, also gold-plated. Wat Pho was established by King Rama III in the 19th century as both a temple and Thailand's foremost university of healing and massage. It still doubles as both, and traditional Thai massage (not a particularly gentle experience) can still be had there.

Some 30 miles (50 kilometers) west of Bangkok is the Phra Pathom Chedi stupa—another of the majestic royal temples. It was built by King Mongkut (Rama IV) on the site of a temple believed to be over 2,000 years old.

A taxiboat waits in the shallows on the beach at Koh Tao for its next fare. Access to many of the islands in the area is by boat only.

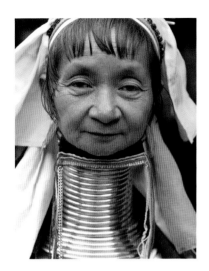

These brass rings adorning a Karen woman are symbols of beauty and status.

With strict antidrug laws, openly smoking in Thailand is extremely unwise.

For a mountain experience you can head for Chiang Mai in the north of the country. This is a jumping-off point for excursions to visit the indigenous highland peoples such as the Karen, Lahu, Hmong, Lisu, Akha, and Mien. The ancient traditions of these "hill tribes" remain very much alive, although the ethnotourism economy in the region has, ironically, led to a degree of cultural erosion.

THE LOWS

Thailand has seen much political unrest in recent years, and some very rowdy protests. Even in the tourist-paradise beaches, there can be a sinister undercurrent. After the devastation of the 2004 tsunami, villagers found their lands seized by armed gunmen in the pay of real-estate speculators.

In Koh Tao it's recommended that tourists keep an eye out for raids by the Maritime Police, who have been known to arrive in a small fleet of boats, conduct searches of cabins, and take in anyone found in possession of cannabis.

If you stick to the islands of the Gulf of Thailand and the Andaman Sea on the other side of the Malay Peninsula (where Phuket is), you won't have to worry too much about the Thai political situation and the current interfactional demonstrations and counterdemonstrations. Anywhere else in the country, you should be aware of some local conflicts. There have been some terrorist attacks in Bangkok in recent years; there is also an ongoing counterinsurgency war in the country's Muslim south, and militarization related to drug enforcement in the opium-growing Golden Triangle in the north.

And while the draconian drug laws are definitely enforced in Bangkok and Chiang Mai, the oppressive sex-tourism trade flourishes with impunity. On the more prosaic side, getting around Bangkok on foot can be hell. There is virtually no way to cross the broad, traffic-clogged thoroughfares.

THE DOPE

There are some skilled cannabis growers along the Gulf of Thailand. The island of Koh Chang (near the Cambodian border) is especially known as a source of ancient cannabis varieties. A perfectly pure sativa known as Wild Thailand is said to have some of the highest THC content of any strain on Earth; its seeds are much sought after by growers around the world.

Reports state that cannabis is cheap and easy enough to come by in Koh Tao. One café at least is known to serve marijuana cake and has a backroom where bongs are filled for consumption on the premises. Bangkok is a slightly more paranoid scene, but cannabis can be found there too in the red-light district. Khao San Road, where backpackers from around the world stay in the cheap hotels, is also a hangout for local dealers.

Dope Sheet

THE PRODUCT: Wild Thailand, a pure sativa, has among the highest THC content of any cannabis in the world; many other less-potent varieties are also grown.

LOOK OUT FOR: Sandy beaches; exceptional wildlife tours at Ang Thong Marine Park; boat trips and snorkeling; the city of Ayutthaya is a World Heritage Site; head to Bangkok and Chiang Mai for temples and palaces, bustling streetlife and lively nightlife.

The pure-sativa Wild Thailand provides a strong, cerebral high.

KNOW THE LAW

Thailand's Narcotics Act is one of the harshest drug laws on earth. You can get long prison terms for possession of even small quantities—and the death penalty for larger quantities of "hard drugs," last enforced in 2004. A few Westerners have been faced with lengthy terms and threat of execution in recent years after getting busted in Thailand—although for heroin and methamphetamine, not cannabis. Tourists busted with cannabis have been known to get off with a fine—after a short stay in jail waiting to see the judge (although "short" can mean several days, not hours). Bail may or may not be offered.

KINGSTON
JAMAICA

Jamaicans were smoking cannabis for at least a century before the Rastafari movement emerged in the 1920s, but what began as a mystical Black nationalist sect has been key to spreading cannabis culture across the planet.

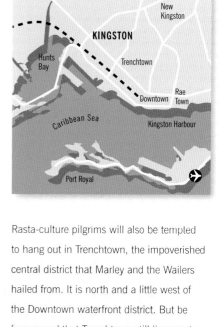

 A mural in tribute to the late Bob Marley, arguably Kingston's most famous son.

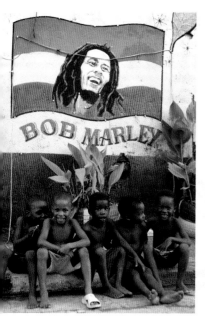

The movement's global icon, Bob Marley, became the first Third World superstar in the 1970s and an international proselytizer of social justice, racial equality, and the sacred herb. A first stop for pilgrims is the Bob Marley Museum at 56 Hope Road, the former office of the Wailers' Tuff Gong record label and now a repository of artifacts and memorabilia of the culture hero's life.

THE HIGHS

Hope Road is a major artery that cuts through the city from the hills in the northeast to the waterfront on the southwest. The current Tuff Gong headquarters is at 220 Marcus Garvey Drive, and it hosts the biggest recording studio in the Caribbean. Record collectors will want to check in to browse the storefront's collection.

Rasta-culture pilgrims will also be tempted to hang out in Trenchtown, the impoverished central district that Marley and the Wailers hailed from. It is north and a little west of the Downtown waterfront district. But be forewarned that Trenchtown still lives up to its tough reputation. Rae Town, along the waterfront east of Downtown, is another center of reggae and Rasta culture, but not quite as edgy as Trenchtown.

Kingston is divided between the old city near the waterfront—including Downtown and Trenchtown—and the more upscale New Kingston inland to the north, where Knutsford Boulevard is the main drag. Which area you want to stay in depends on your budget and how adventurous you are.

Other Kingston tourist draws include Spanish Town on the western outskirts of the city, capital of the island under Spanish rule from

1494 to 1655, when the British took over. The British kept it as the capital until 1872, when it was overtaken by Kingston proper. There's a lot of history here: the notorious pirate Calico Jack Rackham was tried here in 1720; Simón Bolívar plotted the liberation of South America here in 1815; and the proclamation abolishing slavery in Jamaica was read from the Old King's House in 1834. This stately old building is the former residence of Jamaica's British governors. Famous former guests include Captain Bligh of HMS *Bounty* fame and Admiral Horatio Nelson. The Jamaican People's Museum of Crafts and Technology details what life was like for the common people in colonial times. Spanish Town also has a very busy and colorful local market in the central square.

At the old pirate base of Port Royal, once known as the "Sodom of the New World," you can rent scuba gear to check out shipwrecks and the "sunken city" that slipped into the sea in a 1692 earthquake. It is at the end of a long spit of land opposite the Kingston waterfront called the Palisadoes.

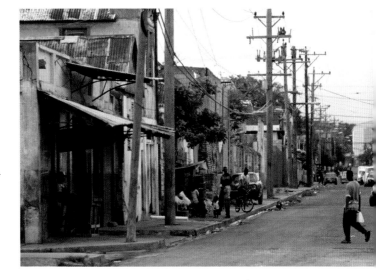

The 50-acre (20-hectare) Hope Botanical Gardens is an oasis in the midst of downtown Kingston, with forest grounds, cactus garden, orchid house, and ornamental pond.

Rising just east of Kingston are the 7,400-foot (2,250-meter) Blue Mountains—famous for both their coffee and ganja. As you ascend, you enter a cool, damp microclimate. You can get a cup of the local "world's best" coffee at the century-old factory in Mavis Bank. There are several fabled "Ganja

Many parts of Kingston are run down; backpackers and travelers should exercise savvy.

Jamaica's Blue Mountains, home to the famous Jamaican Blue Mountain Coffee, also have extensive but well-hidden ganja plantations.

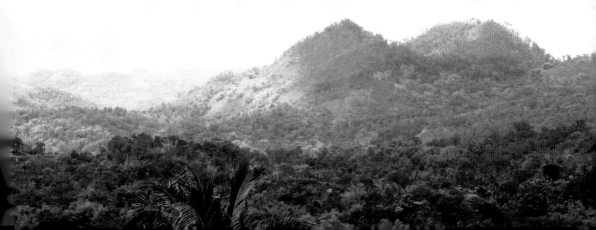

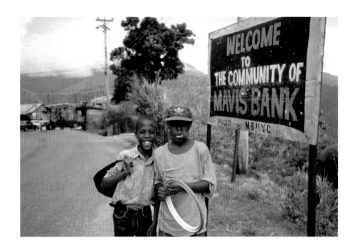

🌿 *Jamaicans in the Blue Mountain town of Mavis Bank. The mountains are frequently shrouded in mist, and hence appear blue.*

🌿 *The first Reggae Sunsplash lasted a marathon seven days.*

those whose interest in herbology extends beyond ganja. The Maroons—runaway slaves who took refuge in these mountains in colonial times—kept alive African traditions and herblore that survive today.

Ocho Rios itself is famous for its reefs and diving. The scenic Dunn's River waterfalls, about 3 miles (5 kilometers) west of Ocho Rios, is another draw for nature-lovers, and there are nearby lodgings that are discreetly ganja-friendly. You can also drive through the verdant Fern Gully, a deep gorge that snakes up into the mountains.

Mountains" up here too, but you'll need to cultivate your own connections to ever see them. For hiking and spectacular views, try Hardwar Gap and John Crow National Park. Bicycle tours of these lush highlands can be arranged out of Ocho Rios, a tourist enclave across the mountains from Kingston on the north coast. There are also "bush medicine" walking tours through the mountains for

Music-lovers will want to time their trip for Reggae Sunsplash, the big summer festival held across the island from Kingston at Montego Bay in the northwest. Held every year since 1978, it features the island's top talent, and today also draws international stars.

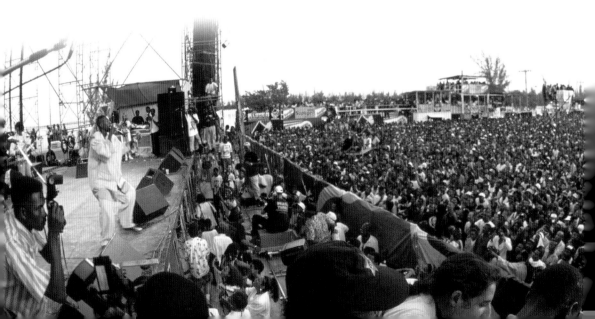

THE LOWS

Inevitably, the mixture of local poverty and global tourism creates a subculture of hustlers and tourist parasites. They can be aggressive, but if you are politely firm you'll be fine. The notorious political violence of the 1970s has largely subsided, but there is still a problem with violent crime. It's good to have some street savvy if you're going to spend any time hanging out in the rougher areas of Kingston.

THE DOPE

Ganja is sold pretty openly on the streets of Rae Town, although to get the better-quality stuff interested parties will have to spend some time making connections. Ganja in Kingston is cheap by Western standards, and elsewhere on the island it is even cheaper. The oldest strains—first brought to the island by immigrants from India in the mid-19th century—are pure sativas. However, in recent years local growers have been hybridizing with seed stock from around the world, and these old Caribbean varieties are disappearing.

Smoking habits are very relaxed in Jamaica. Especially with potent stuff, locals will briefly toke on a single spliff at short intervals for hours, rather than getting blasted in one fell swoop, Western-style. Knowing this, you can avoid etiquette violations when smoking with traditional old-school

Jamaicans. Many Jamaicans also drink ganja tea—to which they attribute various therapeutic and medicinal properties.

KNOW THE LAW

The text of Jamaica's Dangerous Drugs Act endearingly refers to cannabis as "ganja." But the law is not a friendly one—simple possession can lead to a long prison sentence. It seems this generally isn't applied to tourists caught with very small quantities, but this cannot be guaranteed. Enforcement is not too aggressive, and with some common-sense discretion smokers shouldn't have too many problems. Several official commissions have recommended decriminalization, but so far the government has not acted on these results.

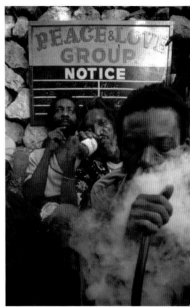

While the local custom is to smoke in moderation over many hours, some prefer a little more immediate relief.

Dope Sheet

THE PRODUCT: The oldest strains of dope are potent pure-sativa, but these are rare; more common are hybrid varieties.

LOOK OUT FOR: The Bob Marley Museum for those on a pilgrimage, along with Trenchtown where he lived; Rae Town for a safer alternative to Trenchtown; head to Marcus Garvey Drive on the waterfront to visit Tuff Gong studio and record shop for a taste of the island's strong musical heritage.

ZIPOLITE
MEXICO

Zipolite Beach on the Pacific coast of Mexico's Oaxaca state is something of a temporary autonomous zone. On the sun-drenched Costa Chica, it is one of Mexico's only nude beaches, and a magnet for free spirits.

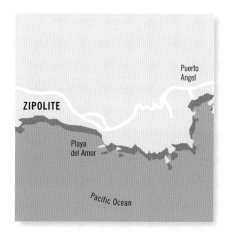

O fficially a self-governing *municipio*, Zipolite has no police force. The volunteer lifeguards—identifiable by their T-shirts emblazoned with "SALVAVIDA OAXACA"—constitute a mellow and de facto constabulary. They have blow-horns and four-wheel drives but no firearms. They are friendly and not at all intimidating. Get to know them, and they'll watch your back.

The small beach community at Zipolite was founded by hippies in the 1970s who had originally camped here to enjoy a solar eclipse.

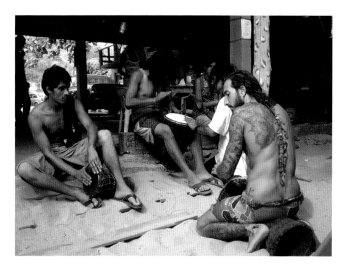

THE HIGHS

The odor of burning buds wafting down the beach is very common. The sun sets into a V-shaped rock outcropping, and watching it with a beer (or what have you) is a ritual each evening—usually followed by a soccer match. On full moons there are rave parties with bonfires and all-night dancing. There are a few secluded areas separated from the main beach by outcroppings, where little communities of transients spring up. The gay section is at the beach's south end. Seafood is fresh, cheap, and tasty.

After being wiped out by 1997's Hurricane Paulina, Zipolite has been rebuilt along slightly more upscale lines, but this is still a budget beach scene with a hippie vibe. At the high end of the spectrum is the Hotel Delfine, which also rents out little cabins called *casitas*. At the other end are campgrounds with *palapas*—little partly enclosed structures, basically a thatch roof supported by a couple of beams where a hammock can be slung. There's no locked door to protect from robbery or mosquitoes, but the price is next to nothing. The campground at La Isla is along a secluded lagoon, and it's run by friendly folks who cook up great fish, rice, and beans each night. Horseback trips along the beach can also be had from here.

Near La Isla is the Iguana Azul nightspot that features techno, reggae, cumbias, and the sounds of Mexican rock bands. A more centrally located nightspot is La Puesta, which strictly features old-school reggae.

There are other great beaches in the immediate area. If you are looking for more of a back-to-nature scene (and to escape from the techno beats), try Mazunte, less than a mile west along the coast. Its economy was long based on harvesting sea-turtle eggs (thought to have aphrodisiac qualities), but happily authorities are now cracking down on this trade, and Mazunte is making the

transition to ecotourism. There is a turtle sanctuary and turtle museum. You're likely to see a turtle in the wild, and the spout of cetaceans is a common sight all along this coast.

A little further in the other direction from Zipolite—across the little town of Puerto Angel to the east—is Estacahuite, famous for its snorkeling. Puerto Angel itself is a good place to hook up with local fishermen if you want to arrange an ocean excursion and see what you can bring in. While there is good surfing at Zipolite, the real surfing scene is at Puerto Escondido, about 40 miles (60 kilometers) up the coast.

When it is winter in Gringolandia, it is blazing on the Costa Chica, and that is the time to go. Be aware that Zipolite is jam-packed at Christmas and Easter, and the price for a hotel room will double. There's a big, seriously crowded, New Year's Eve party on the beach.

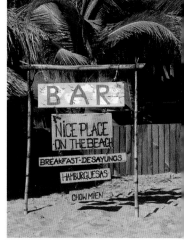

Over the years, the laid-back attitude at Zipolite has attracted backpackers and surfers with a taste for bud.

Following Hurricane Paulina in 1997, much of the community has been rebuilt.

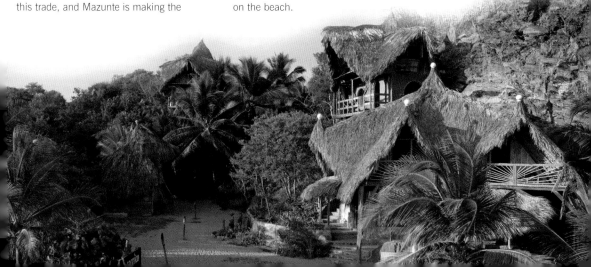

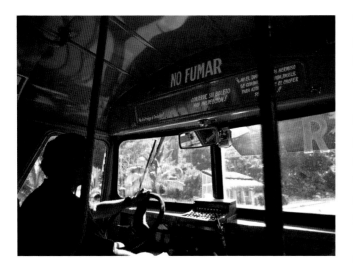

"No Smoking" says the sign on this Mexican bus; a restriction that certainly doesn't hold at Zipolite.

To get to Zipolite, take a bus from Acapulco or Oaxaca City to Pochutla, the nearest town of any size. From there you can get a collectivo microbus to the beach—or at least to Puerto Angel, which is just a 15-minute walk away. Alternatively, you can fly from Mexico City to the big tourist development of Huatulco, some 30 miles (50 kilometers) to the east.

THE LOWS

Rip-offs have long been a problem at Zipolite, and there have been a few rapes and murders over the years. Informal vigilance networks organized by the lifeguards have rolled back the crime somewhat, but nothing can be done about the precarious rip tides that have claimed several lives. By some accounts, the name Zipolite is based on a Nahuatl Indian word meaning

"beach of death." If you are going to swim, pay attention to the flags placed by the lifeguards: green for OK, yellow for caution, and red for dangerous.

In addition to human predators, there are packs of wild dogs that roam the more remote parts of the beach late at night. Stay away from them. And if you walk barefoot, be careful not to step on a spiny sea urchin. It hurts like blazes, and you'll need antibiotics.

On Fridays and Saturdays cops will sometimes come from Pochutla, the nearest town with a police force. They don't really have jurisdiction in Zipolite, but don't try arguing. Keep an eye open for them, and give them a wide berth. Police also frequently search the buses leaving Zipolite—so exporting anything bought on the beach is not recommended.

Unfortunately, smack and coke are also readily available in Zipolite.

THE DOPE

Mexican pot has a reputation as bargain-basement shwag that it has now really outgrown. In the USA, Mexican imports mean dry, compacted brown stuff. This is in large part produced by slave labor in remote mountain areas colonized by the violent cartels. The stuff grown for local consumption by genuine enthusiasts is another story—

fragrant, green buds. There is plenty of fresh Oaxacan on the Costa Chica. Traditionally, Mexican varieties are pure sativa, but indica strains have been making their way down there from California in recent years. What the locals call "Skunky" is widely available. Prices seem to vary according to how long you've been in town and who you know.

KNOW THE LAW

Mexico's current drug code is vague, and gives judges wide discretion to impose fines or prison terms for possession of any controlled substance. Fortunately, this seems about to change, with a groundswell for decriminalization in response to the growing drug-related violence. In 2006, Mexico's Congress passed a bill decriminalizing possession of small amounts of drugs but, following pressure from the US, then-

> # *Dope Sheet*
>
> 🌿 **THE PRODUCT:** The locally grown varieties of Oaxacan are potent; Skunky, an indica-sativa strain is widely available.
>
> 🌿 **LOOK OUT FOR:** Good surfing, but watch out for rip tides; sunsets on the beach; vibrant nightlife, particularly on Fridays and Saturdays; Mazunte turtle sanctuary and museum; good snorkeling can be had at nearby Estacahuite.

President Vicente Fox vetoed it. The current president, Felipe Calderón—who has aggressively deployed the army to fight the cartels—pledged that he would sign such legislation. In April 2009, Congress again approved a decriminalization bill, putting Calderón on the spot. At the time of writing he has yet to sign it.

🌿 *It may look tranquil here, but the beach at Zipolite has claimed many lives; ignore the beach flags at your peril.*

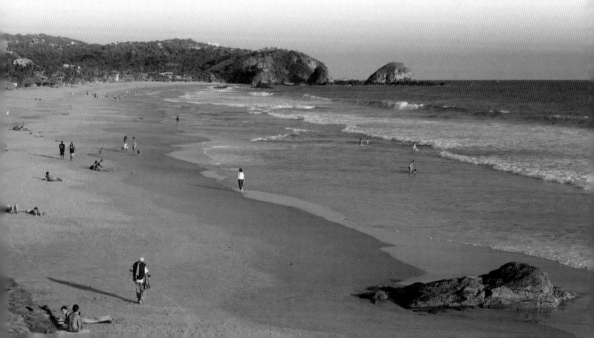

RIO DE JANEIRO
BRAZIL

Brazil's cannabis scene has chilled out considerably since the country decriminalized possession of personal quantities. From the famous Lapa Stairs in Rio to Santa Catarina's beaches, a culture based on marijuana, reggae, and hip-hop is ubiquitous.

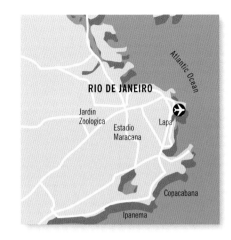

RIO DE JANEIRO

Atlantic Ocean

Jardin Zoologica

Lapa

Estadio Maracana

Copacabana

Ipanema

Brazilians are naturally gregarious. On any night you can go to the Stairs—a large area that borders both downtown and the poor *favelas* (shanty towns)—and mingle with hundreds and sometimes thousands gathered to drink sugar-cane liquor, listen to music, talk, and smoke *maconha* (cannabis).

THE HIGHS

Rio de Janeiro is, of course, one of the most spectacular megalopoli on earth, and it is home to some 14 million people. The Serra da Carioca, a small but steep spur of green mountains sheltered by

Tijuca National Park, cuts through the center of the city, dropping to the downtown district called Centro. It serves as a sort of social barrier, dividing the bourgeois Zona Sul from the working-class districts and favelas of Zona Norte. The two zones meet at Centro.

For magnificent views, take the cable-car to the top of Pão de Açúcar—the iconic Sugarloaf that rises from a peninsula jutting out into the mouth of the bay. Not quite as high but still impressive is Corcovado—the Hunchback—in the Serra da Carioca, crowned by the white statue of Cristo Redentor.

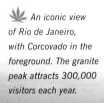
An iconic view of Rio de Janeiro, with Corcovado in the foreground. The granite peak attracts 300,000 visitors each year.

There are great beaches along the coast in both directions—Copacabana and the upscale Ipanema on the shore of Zona Sul being the most famous. Barra da Tijuca, further down the coast from Ipanema at the foot of the mountains, is recommended as at least slightly less crowded and more relaxed as well as providing greener vistas. There is also a hippie hang-out section of Ipanema called (somewhat derisively) the Cemetério dos Elefantes.

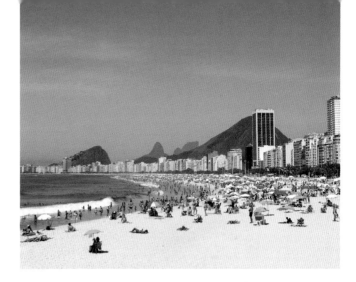

The Flamengo, Glória, and Catete districts, along the waterfront near Centro, are good for cheap lodgings and also convenient for the beaches and sightseeing. Although somewhat run down, there is a sophisticated Art Deco feel to this area, and the Flamengo metro station affords quick access around the city. There's a nearby farmers' market, a public fish market, good Chinese restaurants, juice bars, and a skateboard park.

There's great nightlife all over the city. The high-end Ipanema nightspots are always jumping, but for more of an alternative scene try the Lapa district, just north of Glória. This is the cradle of Brazilian bohemia; the music is more eclectic (acoustic *choros* and experimental electronica as well as frenzied *sambas*) and the conversation more intellectual. The scene is spilling over into the nearby hilltop district of Santa Teresa, which also hosts one of Rio's iconic

attractions, the Arcos de Lapa. Originally a part of the Carioca Aqueduct, the arches now support a tram bridge that connects Santa Teresa hill with Centro. The Lapa Stairs—inlaid in artistic patterns with blue, green, and gold tiles, the colors of the Brazilian flag—go up to one of the funkier parts of Santa Teresa. There's also a cog-rail line.

Rio is transformed into a bacchanalia of samba and chaos every year for Carnival, four days that fall 40 days before Easter. You need a ticket to get into the Sambodromo, the main parade grounds, but the whole city is turned into a party.

For an excursion down the coast, lots of surfers and hippie types head for Garopaba, some 300 miles (500 kilometers) below Rio in Santa Catarina state. The beach there is

Copacabana is just one of many sandy beaches along Rio's stretch of coastline.

The world-famous Rio Carnival started in the 1930s; for four days the entire city turns into the world's biggest street party.

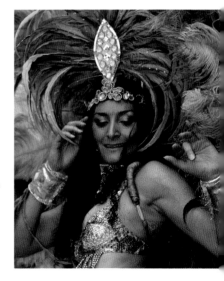

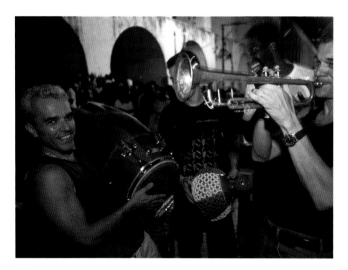

Musicians play samba in the street at Lapa, a bohemian quarter near downtown Rio.

In 2008, the Carnival was marred by deadly violence. As street parties began, police raided some favelas in anti-drug operations that left several dead. At least twenty people were killed in favela raids in 2009. The operations came as officials unveiled a new strategy for a permanent police presence in the favelas rather than withdrawing after shoot-outs. This has been controversial too, however, as many residents view this as a military occupation of their communities.

If you're going to venture into the favelas, it's good to have a trusted connection there. In general, be careful on Rio's streets after dark.

famous for its perfect waves, and marijuana —not always the best quality—is widely available. The population swells to over 100,000 during the Christmas and Carnival holiday seasons, but the rest of the year it is a sleepy beach town. Fishermen and surfers are the only people who stick around all year.

THE LOWS

Urban violence is really at crisis proportions in Rio, and the further north you go in the city the worse it gets. Many of the favelas have been virtually abandoned by the government—except when they send in hundreds of police with machine-guns, armored cars, and helicopters for spectacular drug raids. A 2007 Amnesty International report found that Rio de Janeiro had reached a situation where criminal gangs rushed in to fill the vacuum left by the state, Balkanizing the cities into a patchwork of violent fiefdoms.

THE DOPE

Fresh bud, compressed shwag, and what's locally called *chiba-chiba*—black, gummy, and ultracompressed—are all widely available in Rio. Some is grown locally, but imports from Colombia and Paraguay dominate the market. The most common name for the stuff is maconha, but it is also sometimes *diamba* or *liamba*. These words have their origins in African languages brought to Brazil with slaves from Angola. Especially in the northeast of the country, cannabis has long been used in syncretistic religious rites such as the Catimbó, in which African ceremonial traditions survive.

If you want to meet local tokers in Rio, just head for the Lapa Stairs any evening.

Be aware that phraseology is not too advanced in the local cannabis scene; any good bud will often be called "hydro," even if it is obviously not hydroponic.

Unfortunately, cocainc is much morc frccly available than cannabis in Brazil. In the favelas, both are openly sold at distribution points called *bocas del fumo* (mouths of smoke). But—once again—it is wise to stay out of the favelas without a reliable and knowledgeable connection.

KNOW THE LAW

In 2006, President Luis Inacio "Lula" da Silva signed a decriminalization bill that instates "social education" sentences—community service and "rehabilitation" programs—instead of jail time for those busted with "small quantities" of drugs. What exactly constitutes a "small quantity" is left to the discretion of the judge, but in practice it is about a gram or two of cannabis. The law also increases the minimum prison term for those accused of dealing. The "social education" sentences seem rarely to be enforced for cannabis, however, and especially not for tourists.

Dope Sheet

🌿 **THE PRODUCT:** Most bud is imported from Colombia and Paraguay, although some is locally grown; "chiba-chiba" is sticky and ultracompressed.

🌿 **LOOK OUT FOR:** One of liveliest cities in the world; superb beaches; take the cable-car to Páo de Açúcar for spectacular views; Flamengo, Glória, and Catete for cheap accommodation and Art Deco vibe; fish and farmers' markets; Lapa district for street musicians and bohemian atmosphere.

🌿 *A raid at a slum dwelling in Rocinha, Rio, unearths a cocaine laboratory together with heavy weapons and ammunition.*

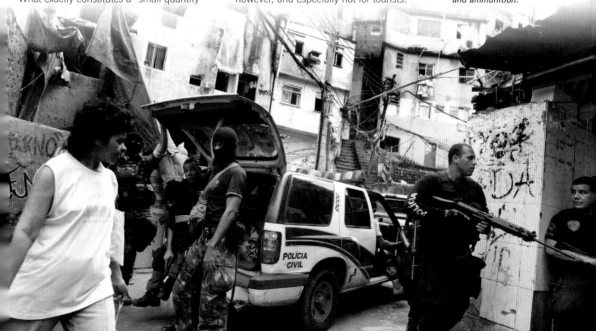

VANCOUVER
CANADA

Vancouver is situated on a magnificent peninsula in the delta of the Fraser River. The snow-capped peaks of the Coast Mountains are just inland, green Vancouver Island is just across the Strait of Georgia to the west, and the views are spectacular.

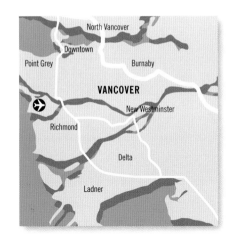

It is also the most cannabis-friendly city in Canada, and, of course, the coffeeshop scene there is becoming known as "Vansterdam"—the center of which is the 300 block of West Hastings Street in the historic Gastown district near the harbor front.

THE HIGHS

Known to locals simply as the "Block," the area was badly damaged by a fire in 2004 but is still going strong. The old Blunt Brothers café burned down but has reopened as the New Amsterdam Café, right next door to the British Colombia Marijuana Party Bookstore.

In July 2009, activist Dana Larsen organized the city's first Vansterdam Ganja Games and Marijuana Bowl, and pledged to make it an annual affair. The three-day extravaganza included a boat cruise and workshops in glassblowing and hash making as well as tasting and rating the latest strains of BC Bud.

Bordering Gastown on the east is Chinatown, one of the biggest in North America. The Commercial Drive district east of Chinatown includes Da Kine Café, which houses the Canadian Sanctuary Society medical-marijuana organization. The nearby Melting

A view across Vancouver with the Coast Mountains in the background.

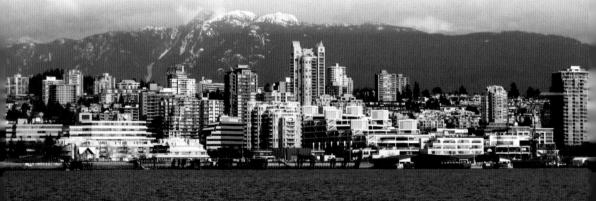

Point store offers vaporizers and hashish-making technology. Both are on the 1000 block of Commercial Drive.

Kitsilano, west of Granville Street, was Vancouver's hippie haven in the 1960s, and the neighborhood still hosts lots of bookstores, restaurants, and cafés. Sativa Sisters Kind Sanctuary Bed and Breakfast in this area is an obvious place to stay and is a short walk from the beach.

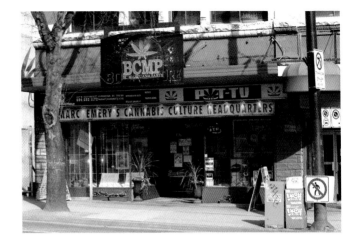

THE LOWS

While Canada is one of the world's safest countries, Vancouver, a major entrepôt for all kinds of contraband, has gained some notoriety for gunplay in recent years. There have been some 500 killed in street turf wars over the past decade, chiefly among the city's Mexican and Asian gangs that control (and fight over) the drug networks.

If you are crossing the US–BC border by car and you have dreadlocks or other such manifestations of the "drug-user" profile, it is quite likely you will be searched.

THE DOPE

Hydroponic BC Bud is fast acquiring legendary status. The strains are largely based on the sativa-indica hybrids that came up from California a generation ago, but local growers have now imported seed stock from all over the world. New strains are always

being developed, and their potency has sparked a media frenzy as more of the stuff has been making it to Canada's east and to stateside markets. A representative of the US Border Patrol has described BC Bud as a "very lethal type of hydroponically grown marijuana." A lawman using the term "lethal" to describe cannabis with a (presumably) straight face indicates how far out of whack the drug-war debate has veered.

KNOW THE LAW

Since 2002, when the Coalition of Progressive Electors gained a majority on the city council, Vancouver has had a tolerant drug policy based on a "harm reduction" model that de-emphasizes enforcement. However, you can still get busted for public smoking, so even at the coffeeshops, feel things out and be discreet. Smoke on the street at your own risk.

🌿 *The headquarters of pro-cannabis supporter Marc Emery.*

🌿 *The suggestively named New Amsterdam Café is in the burgeoning Vansterdam district.*

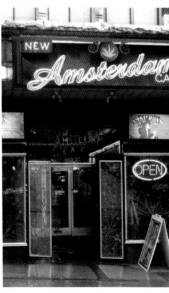

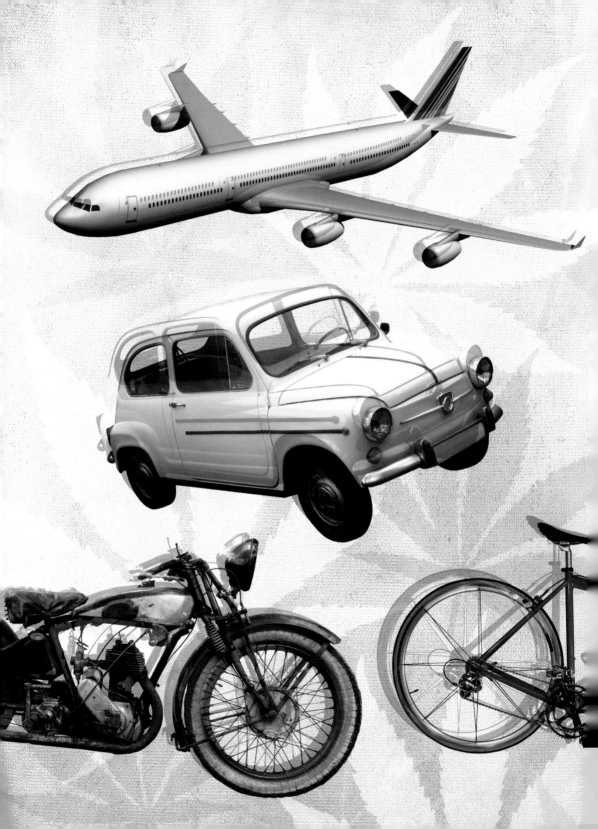

HEAVY TRIPS

There's intrepid and there's downright dangerous, but of course it's your call. The trouble is that some of the most fascinating and beautiful places on earth are also among the most dangerous due to war, crime, poverty, or repression. And that's just to visit, let alone going with a view to searching out the local pot scene. There are some very scary places in this world, so please be forewarned and proceed at your own risk.

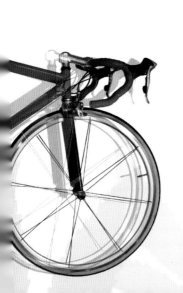

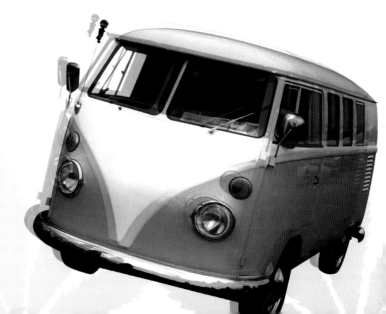

SMOKING GUNS IN COLOMBIA

The really surreal thing about the legal status of cannabis in Colombia is that possessing small quantities of it has been decriminalized since 1994—in a society which in nearly every other way is a right-wing authoritarian state.

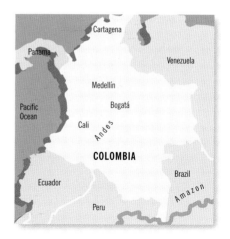

I n the county's second city of Medellín, youth gather nightly in Parque Periodista (literally, Journalist Park) and light up openly, pass bottles around, strum guitars, or blast raps and cumbias from boom boxes. The police are nowhere to be seen and the party goes on long into the night. Yet the country has long been in the grip of right-wing paramilitary groups, whose reign of terror has not ended with the supposed "demobilization" that started in 2003. While they wipe out suspected sympathizers of Colombia's leftist guerilla movements, in their orbit are skinhead gangs who carry out brutal "social cleansing" against gays, peaceniks, punks, and dope-smokers.

This tranquil panoramic view just outside Pasto, southwest Colombia, belies the bloody conflict being constantly waged between the country's various political factions.

THE HIGHS

Colombia is by no means just a bad trip, however. It is the most ecologically and culturally diverse country in South America. It has some of the continent's best music— from the rocking *vallenatas* of the northern mountains to the polyrhythmic *mapalé* of the Afro-Colombian zone along the Caribbean coast. The jungles of Chocó on the Pacific coast are another Afro-Colombian heartland, where elements of African languages survive in the music and culture. Inland from the jungle coastal plain, the Andes rise. This is where the Andean culture that extends all the way down to Chile begins. Across the mountains and south of the eastern plains

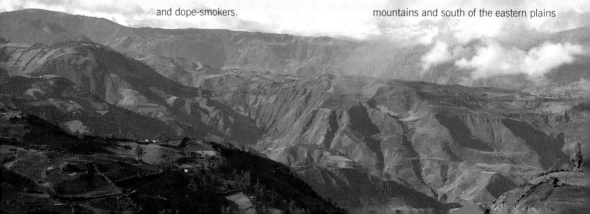

lies the Amazon rainforest, covering a quarter of the country—a vast, sparsely inhabited expanse where the only transportation is bush plane or riverboat, and indigenous shamanic cultures still survive.

In 1994, Colombia's top court ruled that small quantities of illegal drugs were not criminal offenses, and so Colombia joined the Netherlands, Italy, and Spain in decriminalizing. Despite attempts to reverse this subsequently, possession of small quantities remains de facto legal.

The political violence that has plagued the country for decades (see right) has largely scared off the tourists, so Colombia offers a rare taste of unpackaged authenticity. The warmth and gratitude of proud Colombians, who will beam at you for having the courage to visit their country, can be touching.

Colombia has a lot to offer the adventurous traveler, and the fact that it is off the tourist trail makes it that much more real. And, for the toker, in a country where assassinations and kidnappings are near-daily fare, it is possible to smoke cannabis openly and unmolested in a public park. It should be noted that public smoking is not generally tolerated (Parque Periodista is a special "free zone"); but where personal use is concerned, Colombia's policy is far more relaxed than many Western countries.

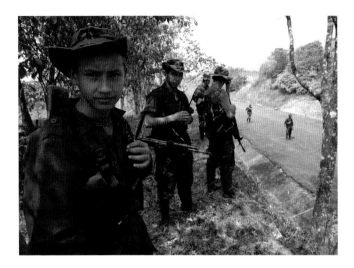

THE LOWS

Travel is dangerous in Colombia, and all the more so if you have a US passport. The army, paramilitaries, and guerillas all set up checkpoints where they stop and search traffic on the roads between the major cities. People are known to disappear at these checkpoints. Foreigners, and Colombians who can afford it, generally fly between cities—and this can get expensive. Many rural areas are war zones—the Amazon region is especially dangerous, but no part of the country is immune from political and drug-related violence.

🌿 *A checkpoint held by young guerilleros from the Colombian Revolutionary Armed Forces (FARC).*

🌿 *Colombia is home to amazingly diverse cultural groups. These children are Nukak Amerindian refugees who have been forced from their land in Colombia's Amazon Basin.*

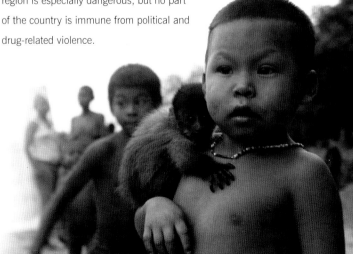

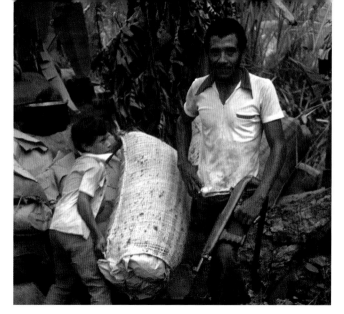

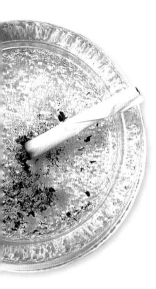

A man guards a marijuana crop with a submachine gun, while a small boy carries a sack of grass off to be loaded.

The cocaine cartels long collaborated with the paramilitaries against the guerillas, basically because the FARC imposed taxes on coca grown in their areas of control, and the cartels wanted a free-trade zone under their exclusive control. When Colombia's National Police and the DEA jointly crushed the drug cartels in the 1990s, this merely set off a new, bloody scramble for mastery over the country's dope trade—this time between the AUC and FARC. Both have massacred peasants who sold coca leaf to the other side.

Crime is rampant in the cities. Hold ups, street scams, and pickpocketing are all organized by serious professionals who are very good at what they do. Sometimes they have a forged police ID; sometimes it isn't forged.

Although best known around the world for its cocaine these days, Colombia still grows loads of cannabis, both for export and internal consumption. The drug cartels first emerged as marijuana syndicates in the 1970s, but in the 1980s these morphed into the cocaine cartels; ever more of the countryside turned to coca cultivation and, later, opium. Currently the various guerilla and paramilitary organizations—most notably the leftist Colombian Revolutionary Armed Forces (FARC) and the ultra-right United Colombian Self-Defense Forces (AUC)—are locked in a struggle for control of the country's coca-growing regions.

Just to make it more bizarre, even as the government has decriminalized personal possession of illegal drugs, it continues to spray the herbicide glyphosate over the country's mountains and jungles to wipe out coca leaf. This spraying is actually done by the private outfit DynCorp in planes directly contracted by the US State Department. The Colombian National Police usually come along for the ride in accompanying helicopters. Peasants have repeatedly complained that their legal crops of corn and beans have been wiped out by the spraying—and even that they have been directly sprayed, causing respiratory problems and ugly rashes.

To wrap up: If you are planning on going to Colombia, be ready for some action. This is not a trip to be taken lightly.

THE DOPE

Known locally as *maracachafa*, *marimba*, and *perico*, marijuana is pretty ubiquitous in Colombia. It's also increasingly known by the Mexican slang term *mota*. It is easy to meet local tokers and dealers. One account on a website boasts of buying a "potato sack filled with red point for about 150 bucks," but this fellow had to go out to the countryside and deal directly with the farmer. Be forewarned: a potato sack filled with weed is definitely not considered a personal quantity! If you get caught with that, be assured of having to pay a very hefty bribe or winding up in Colombia's violence-plagued jails.

And keep in mind that cannabis—while a distant third to coca and opium—is a goad of war in Colombia. As an example, in February 2008, some twenty FARC guerillas were killed in clashes with the army at the village of Chaparral in mountainous Tolima department. High casualties were reportedly due to aerial bombardment of rebel positions by Colombian warplanes. National Police also announced the confiscation of several tons of marijuana that had allegedly belonged to the local FARC column. In other words, it looks as if the Colombian Air Force was bombing marijuana growers, who (willingly or not) had been dealing with the FARC. Just an example of what life is like in Colombia's dope-growing zones.

Dope Sheet

🍁 **THE PRODUCT:** Punto Rojo (or red point) is a highly potent pure sativa variety; Colombian Gold is also a strong variety; it may take time, however, to find either.

🍁 **LOOK OUT FOR:** Candelaria (Old Town) of Bogotá; the historic town of Cartagena; many festivals, including Pasto's Carnival of Blacks and Whites; numerous national parks for ecotourism; either go to the coast, the jungle, or up in the mountains.

🍁 *A soldier from the Colombian army advances in a field of coca while a plane in the background sprays pesticides.*

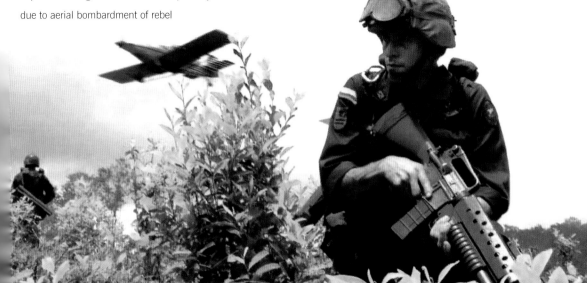

SEVERED HEADS IN MICHOACÁN

Imagine the scene. The crowd is happily dancing, the tequila and beer are flowing. Suddenly, gunmen burst into the bar and seal off the exits. One of them holds a big bag. He reaches in, pulls out five human heads and hurls them on to the dance floor.

A sidewalk produce vendor makes a fruit salad consisting of papaya, jicama, melon, and lime in San Lorenzo, Michoacán.

This is exactly what happened in September 2006 at the Luz y Sombra nightclub in the town of Uruapan, in the Mexican state of Michoacán. The assailants—some wearing police uniforms—also left a message scrawled on a cardboard placard: "The Family doesn't kill for money. It doesn't kill women and it doesn't kill the innocent. Only those who deserve it die. Let it be known: This is divine justice." La Familia—Michoacán's reigning, cultish crime machine—had announced its presence to the world.

THE HIGHS

A particular tragedy of the Michoacán nightmare is that the state is a beautiful one that holds a special place in the heart of Mexicans. For gringo stoners, it has long been synonymous with the higher end of imported Mexican cannabis. For Mexicans, it means a beautiful and (until recently) tranquil vacation destination.

Pine forest covers the mountains. The state's real jewel is Lake Pátzcuaro, west of Morellia, where a 130-foot (40-meter) statue of the independence hero José Maria Morelos rises from Janitzio Island. You can climb up to an observation room in his raised fist for panoramic vistas. The Purépecha Indians fish on the lake, and the trout is delicious.

Continuing west, Uruapan is a center of pottery craftsmanship and avocado cultivation. Nearby is Paricutín Volcano, where you can see the remains of a village that was destroyed by an eruption in 1943, half-buried in solidified lava. You can also take a donkey-back tour of the slope and crater with an Indian guide. It is an eerie moonlike landscape, with life still reemerging from the lava desert.

North of Uruapan, the little town of Paracho is called Mexico's "guitar capital," with hundreds of shops where traditional craftsmen make fine acoustic guitars. The craft is passed down within families from generation to generation, and the guitars are prized across Mexico.

In the mountains to the east of Morelia, the state capital, the Mariposa Monarca Biosphere Reserve is the monarch butterfly's primary wintering ground, and millions of the brightly colored critters converge there from across North America between November and April. And Morelia itself is a beautiful colonial city, looking like it was frozen in time in the 16th century. The historic center is a UN World Heritage Site.

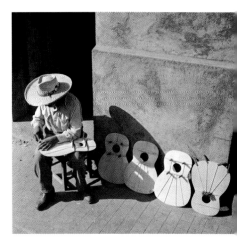

THE LOWS

Beheadings were already a pattern by the time of the Luz y Sombra outrage in Uruapan. In July 2006, in Tepalcatepec, the tortured body of a suspected hitman turned up on the outskirts of town. More would follow. In October, two severed heads were found outside a car showroom in the town of Zitacuaro. The bodies were found several miles away.

Since then the drug wars have escalated. In September 2008, assailants lobbed grenades through the crowded town square in Morelia during Mexican Independence Day

🌿 *The guitars made in Paracho are all hand-crafted and considered the best in Mexico.*

🌿 *Janitzio is one of seven islands on Lake Pátzcuaro, and is inhabited almost entirely by indigenous Purépecha Indians, of which an estimated 200,000 live in Michoacán.*

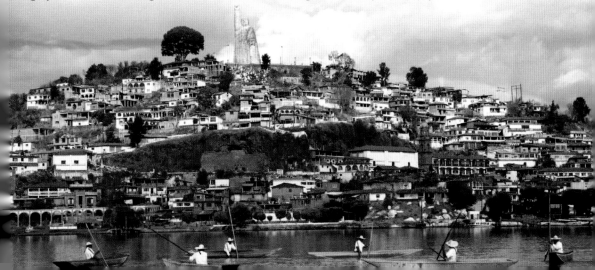

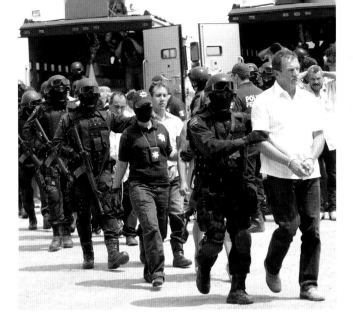

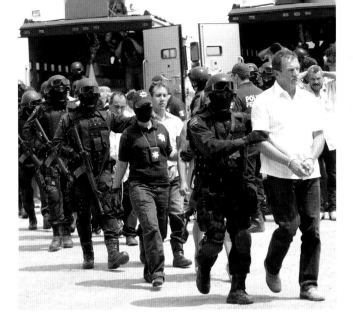 Mexican policemen escort alleged members of the "La Familia Michoacana" drug cartel in Mexico City following a police operation in April 2009.

🌿 Climbers dot the crater rim of Volcán Paricutín, a 10,400-foot (3,100 meter) volcano in Michoacán. A trek to the top is a day-long hike from the Purépecha Indian village of Angahuan.

celebrations. Seven were killed and more than a hundred injured. Suspects were arrested, but the narcos continued to carry out brazen attacks on security forces and each other. By the spring of 2009, La Familia was leaving threatening messages on the bodies of their victims. These were mostly aimed at Los Zetas, the paramilitary arm of the Gulf Cartel, based in the northern border city of Matamoros. La Familia, who study a "special Bible" and claim to be evangelical Christians, started out as a supposed anti-drug vigilante group but are today believed to be allied with the Beltran Leyva crime family—itself a faction of the splintered Sinaloa Cartel. They appear to be defending Michoacán's drug trade from Gulf Cartel encroachment.

In July 2009, the situation escalated towards an actual war on the state. Gunmen tossed grenades and opened fire on Mexican federal police bases and checkpoints in Morelia and in five other Michoacán towns immediately after the arrest of Arnoldo Rueda Medina, AKA "La Minsa," an accused high-ranking Familia jefe (boss). In Apatzingán, assailants shot up a hotel where federal agents were staying. Five federal police agents and two soldiers were killed. The attacks especially targeted towns where federal police arrested local mayors in May that year in an unprecedented sweep of politicians accused of protecting the narcos.

Later, in July, Mexican federal agents detained ten municipal police from Arteaga for the torture and slaying of 12 federales whose bodies were found dumped along a highway. Prosecutors also charged a former mayor of the town of La Huacana, where the mutilated bodies were found.

Also that month, a man claiming to be Familia leader Servando Gómez, AKA "La Tuta," called into a local TV talk show. He said he was attacking security forces simply to defend his followers' families and friends, and proposed talks with the government.

President Felipe Calderón has deployed some 5,500 federal police and army troops to Michoacán to combat La Familia. The left-opposition bloc in the Mexican Senate issued a statement denouncing what it called the illegal and unconstitutional "occupation" of Michoacán, accusing Calderón of attempting to turn it into a "totalitarian state."

And the Mexican security forces have indeed been implicated in some horrific abuses in Michoacán. In 2006, Mexico's National Human Rights Commission confirmed that soldiers had raped at least two underage girls and possibly two others during an anti-drug operation in the village of Caracuaro. Also that year, three lawyers being held hostage by inmates who had lost a court appeal were killed when police raided the state prison at Mil Cumbres.

As a tourist you will come across military and police checkpoints on the roads. If they think you are carrying drugs they will search your vehicle, and if they think they can hit you up for a bribe, they may plant drugs. If this isn't intimidating enough, the likelihood of bullets flying at these roadblocks as they are attacked by narco gunmen is increasing all the time.

Dope Sheet

🌿 **THE PRODUCT:** Potent, sativa-rich bud is readily available; quality is assured by the small independent farmers.

🌿 **LOOK OUT FOR:** Lake Pátzcuaro; pottery at Uruapan; Paricutín Volcano for hiking and the remains of a half-buried village; the attractive colonial city of Morelia; Paracho, the guitar-capital of Mexico; head for Mariposa Monarca Biosphere Reserve to see millions of overwintering monarch butterflies.

THE DOPE

It is everywhere, and it is good, strong sativa. This was Mexico's heartland of marijuana cultivation for generations before the cartels established their big slave-labor plantations in the Sierra Madre of Chihuahua and Durango states to the north. Michoacán still grows plenty of Mexico's finest. Much of it is still cultivated by small independent peasant growers—and distributed by networks with at least some degree of independence from the ultraviolent cartels. The real local lucre is in the cocaine trade.

🌿 *A US surfer on vacation proudly displays a handful of potent mota.*

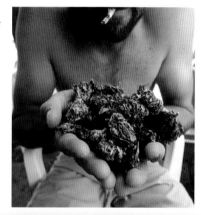

Toking in War Zones

Here's the scariest thing that's ever happened to me in all my life.

In 1985, I was a hippie vagabond with a ponytail and a mandolin on the road in Central America. I was attracted by the romance of the revolutionary movements then active in the isthmus, but I also wanted to visit beautiful places, get high, and have fun. In tranquil Belize I smoked spliffs on Maya ruins with local rastas. Then, I crossed the jungle border into Guatemala—and decided to venture into some very dangerous territory.

Guatemala at that time was under a military dictatorship that was carrying out a campaign of genocide against the country's indigenous Maya peoples. I had heard stories of the mountain hamlets burned, the inhabitants massacred or forced to flee, and those left relocated into military-controlled "model villages"—very nearly concentration camps. I wanted to know what it was like. I took the bus right through the most militarized part of the Maya Highlands. At sundown, we arrived at the village of Uspantán, where there was a brief stopover. I decided to go for a walk. I took my mandolin and wandered up the dirt road into the mountains, figuring to catch the last of the twilight, maybe play a hornpipe or two under a tree, and then head back. Big mistake.

The next thing I knew, a posse carrying old carbine rifles was approaching me, surrounding me, leveling their guns at me. One relieved me of my mandolin; another took out a rope and tied my hands behind me. Then they marched me with a rifle in my back up the mountain— *away from town*. By this point it began to dawn on me what had happened. This was the Civil Patrol—Indians deputized by the military as an anti-guerilla vigilante force. They were enforcing a dusk curfew. The patrol marched me up the road to a camp and put me in a bamboo cage with my wrists tied to the bars and their rifles all trained on me.

My first dumb concern was that the bus was going to leave without me. Then, it hit me—I would disappear into the clandestine prisons of Guatemala. I could face torture or death. I would never see friends or family again. Soon enough, the

🌿 *Guatemala's Civil Patrols were paramilitary groups set up by the government to fight in the countryside.*

local army guy who oversaw the Civil Patrol arrived at the camp. He opened my mandolin case, and I was relieved to see him actually smile when he saw it was just a mandolin inside. I was overawed at my own stupidity. When he approached me, I played (without having to pretend too much) the dumb tourist. I told him the embarrassing truth, that I'd been sightseeing and didn't know there was a curfew and had a bus to catch. Much to my relief, he believed me, and with a sinister sense of false camaraderie, he ordered me released. The next day I left for the Mexican border. I'd had enough of Guatemala.

Guatemala is at peace today, and Lake Atitlán especially is a hippie destination. I tell this story to illustrate the dangers of being a happy-go-lucky vagabond in a war zone. I'm lucky I didn't get shot. If I hadn't kept my wits, it could have turned ugly at any moment. If they'd found pot in my mandolin case, the story could have had a very different ending.

Cannabis is mixed up with warfare in much of the world. Ten years after my Guatemalan escapade, I went, as a journalist for *High Times* magazine, to Chiapas in southern Mexico to cover the army's supposed marijuana-eradication operations, which were actually aimed at establishing a military presence on lands sympathetic to the Zapatista rebels. (This was a way of getting around an official truce that had been brokered.) Meanwhile, the stuff was actually grown by pro-government peasants who organized paramilitary groups to terrorize Zapatista sympathizers.

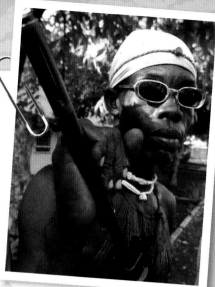

The Kamajor militia are rebels who later joined forces with the Sierra Leonean government in their war against the RUF.

Teun Voeten, a Belgian photographer whom I worked with in Mexico and Central America in those years, would later spend time in the war-torn West African nation of Sierra Leone, where he covered the demobilization of child soldiers, and was trapped as a ceasefire broke down. In his memoir of his harrowing escape he relates how the Revolutionary United Front (RUF) used *jamba* (cannabis) as well as amphetamines to disorientate and indoctrinate abducted children and turn them into killers.

In many spots, cannabis eradication and counterinsurgency are thoroughly entwined. The southern Philippine island of Mindanao is said to have great marijuana—but the government claims it is grown by the Abu Sayyaf militant group, and those busted for cultivation or even possession fall under suspicion of terrorism as well.

If you're going to be toking in war zones, understand the risks, beware of compromising situations—and have a sense of how cannabis affects your own emotional reactions to danger. Only you can determine this, and having a realistic idea could literally save your life.

FLOGGED FOR HASH IN AFGHANISTAN

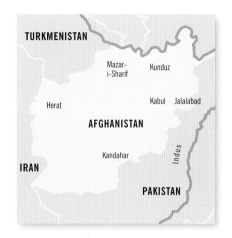

Considering that the Taliban have been known to stone women to death for "adultery" (which can include being raped), you could say they mollycoddle hashish smokers. Normally they are only publicly flogged.

In their years in power from 1996 to 2001, the Taliban's Ministry for the Promotion of Virtue and Prevention of Vice oversaw punishments that conformed to their ultraorthodox interpretation of Sharia law. After the US-led invasion of November 2001, a reporter examined records seized from this agency of fear. One entry he found referred to a local resident being "addicted to hashish"; the man was sentenced to be whipped with a 5-inch (13-centimeter)-wide leather strap known as a *dura*.

An Afghan tribesman surveys southeastern Kabul from one of the hills that surround the town.

THE HIGHS

The hippies, seekers, and cannabis enthusiasts who came to Afghanistan on the "Overland Trail" from India and Pakistan in the late 1960s and early 1970s didn't know how lucky they were. This was actually one of the few brief windows of opportunity in history when it was possible for outsiders to visit the country. In "My Summer Vacation in Afghanistan," an essay written at the time of the US invasion, Peter Lamborn Wilson recalled his 1969 arrival from Iran:

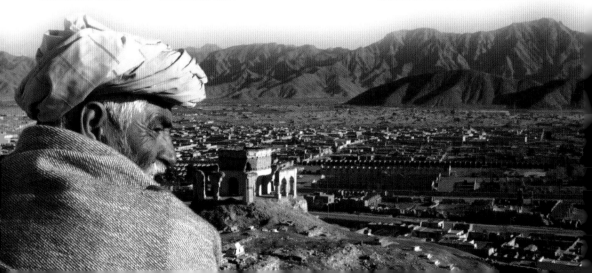

"Crossing the border, an Afghan guard entered the bus, which was full of hippies: '*Any you got hashish?*' he screamed. Chorus of '*No,*' '*No,*' '*Not me,*' '*Not me, sir*'—squeaky and scared. What the hell? '*Sssooo...*' hissed the officer, reaching menacingly into his jacket, '*you like to buy?*' He whipped out a chunk of hash the size of a loaf of Wonder Bread. '*Very good, grade-A Afghani.*'"

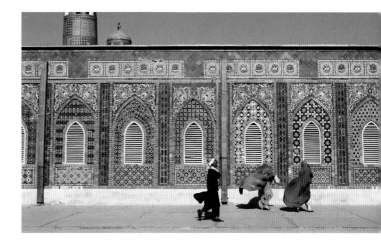

It is uncertain if the window is opening again two generations later. Western dreams of installing a stable democracy in Afghanistan look increasingly dubious, and central-government control is nonexistent in many parts of the country. If you do make it, however, there is a circuit you can do of Afghanistan's cities—each one of them a historic treasure.

From Kabul—a city largely destroyed by a generation and more of war—first head southwest along the Pashtun belt to Kandahar, where Taliban sympathies run deepest. If you make it there intact, you can see the magnificent Mausoleum of Ahmed Shah Durrani, the father of Afghanistan, who reigned from 1747 to 1772. Nearby is the Shrine of the Cloak of the Prophet, which by local lore holds the robe worn by the Prophet Mohammed. The city was founded by Alexander the Great, and its name is a corruption of "Alexander."

From Kandahar the road bends in a long arc to the north toward Herat, where the population are mostly ethnic Persians. In the north, you are leaving behind the Taliban insurgency; now you only have to worry about bandits and freebooting warlords. If you make it to Herat alive, you can see the shrine of Khwaja Abdullah Ansaru, the 11th-century Sufi saint.

From here the road turns northeast into the Uzbek heartland of Mazar-i-Sharif, domain of the notoriously brutal warlord Abdul Rashid Dostum. Mazar is home to the 15th-century Shrine of Hazrat Ali, which supposedly holds the remains of Islam's fourth caliph. Thousands of pilgrims gather here for the Nowruz spring festival in March. Just before Mazar, you can stop in Balkh and see the shrine of Khwaja Abu Nasr Parsa, another Sufi saint, also dating to the 15th-century Timurid Empire founded by

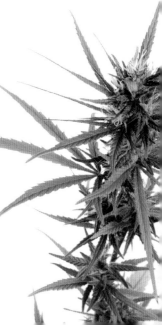

The Shrine of Hazrat Ali, or the Blue Mosque, is said to be the resting place of the fourth caliph. As its alternative name suggests, the Shrine is decorated primarily in blue mosaic tiles.

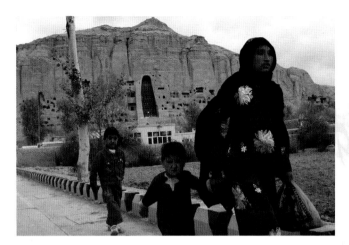

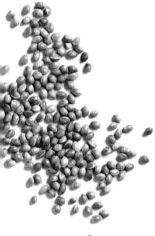

A woman and her children walk along a road in Bamiyan. In the background is visible the now empty niche that once housed a 174-foot (53-meter) Buddha, destroyed by the Taliban in 2001.

the famous Uzbek-Mongol conqueror Tamerlane, or Timur-i-Leng. Also in Balkh is the 9th-century Masjid-e-Noh Gumbad, the earliest Islamic monument in Afghanistan.

Continuing east from Mazar, you may be fortunate enough to arrive still breathing at Kunduz, where the road turns south into Tajik territory and brings you back to Kabul.

If you come in from Pakistan via the Khyber Pass, you can stop in Jalalabad, where ancient Buddhist stupas have somehow survived both Soviet bombardment and Taliban defacement. There was a unique Greco-Buddhist civilization in Afghanistan for some 500 years from around 100 BCE. Unfortunately, the giant stone Buddhas at Bamiyan in the remote central mountains of the Hindu Kush—Afghanistan's most precious heritage to humanity—were destroyed by the Taliban in March 2001.

THE LOWS

With no sign of any resolution to the ongoing conflict, these should be obvious. The terse warning of the US State Department insists that "no part of Afghanistan should be considered immune from violence, and the potential exists throughout the country for hostile acts, either targeted or random, against American and other Western nationals at any time."

Outside of Kabul, electricity is sporadic at best. Dust is everywhere. Women throughout Afghanistan are expected to wear the full-body covering known as the burqa, or at least the face covering called a chador. In Kabul, exceptions may be made for foreigners.

Practices such as stoning for adultery were supposedly abolished after the fall of the Taliban, but, in fact, they continue. In 2005 a woman was dragged from her parents' home by the "official" police, buried up to the waist, and stoned to death by a mob following an order from a local court. The man she was accused of committing adultery with got off with a hundred lashes. This kind of act is not confined to rural areas. In 2004, two European travelers, who had just arrived from Pakistan, were stoned to death in Kabul—Afghanistan's capital. Nobody was arrested, and it was never determined what their transgression was. *You have been warned.*

THE DOPE

Cannabis has traditionally been a pillar of the economy in Afghanistan. Travelers in the 1960s and 1970s were attracted by the promise of green-gold Afghani and the tea houses that hosted a hash bazaar in Balkh.

The real hash experience is *charas*, handmade and usually coming in sticks or balls. However, it is harder to find today than 40 years ago, and asking around could make you a target.

Cannabis production has ebbed and flowed with the tides of war. It was banned along with opium by the Taliban. Production of both surged after the Taliban fell. Now that they are out of power, there are indications that they are turning to the opium trade to fund their insurgency. A US-backed campaign is making some headway against opium, but lots of farmers are just switching to cannabis.

Dope Sheet

THE PRODUCT: Historically the sought-after hash was charas, which was available in balls or sticks.

LOOK OUT FOR: Kabul, although now largely destroyed; the Mausoleum of Ahmed Shah Durrani and the Shrine of the Cloak of the Prophet in Kandahar; the Shrine of Hazrat Ali in Mazar-i-Sharif; the ancient Buddhist stupas at Jalalabad.

US and Afghan soldiers and Afghan National Police officers question a farmer after finding a field full of marijuana plants.

A 2006 CNN report noted that Canadian troops fighting Taliban insurgents stumbled across impenetrable forests of ten-foot (three-meter) marijuana plants. They tried burning them, initially with no success. But when an area of the crop actually did catch fire, some soldiers were reported to suffer "ill effects," and the attempt was abandoned. Some of the "affected" soldiers may not have agreed with this course of action!

TEN YEARS FOR
A JOINT **IN KENYA**

Kenya's harsh drug laws briefly made world news shortly after US President Barack Obama was inaugurated. His estranged half-brother, George Obama, was arrested just then for possession of one joint in Nairobi.

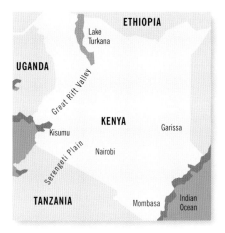

He denied the charge, and it was dropped a couple of days later when the police apparently decided the stuff belonged to some friends arrested along with him. Under Kenyan law, he could have faced anything between ten and twenty years in prison—possibly the folks busted with George did face such harsh terms.

THE HIGHS

The famous game parks are the biggest tourist draw in Kenya. Amboseli, Lake Nakuru, Masai Mara, Meru, and Mt. Kenya national parks are teeming with elephants, giraffes, wildebeest, zebras, antelopes, cheetahs, and lions. To visit most of them, you have to have your own vehicle or join a tour. You can also arrange guides in Nairobi for a trek to the peak of Mt. Kilimanjaro, which rises 15,100 feet (4,600 meters) from the Serengeti Plain on the Tanzanian border.

Kenya's premier cultural event is the Storymoja Hay Festival, which takes place from late July to early August at the Impala Grounds in Nairobi. A celebration of oral folklore and legend, in 2009 it featured Nobel Laureates Wole Soyinka and Wangari Mathai along with other prominent writers, poets, and traditional storytellers. Bands from throughout East Africa provide nightly entertainment at the festival.

Wildebeest are the most common animal found in the Masai Mara Game Reserve.

THE LOWS

Under a 1994 revision of the Narcotic Drugs and Psychotropic Substances Control Act, possession of any quantity of cannabis carries a ten-year term—or, if the judge determines it was intended for sale, a twenty-year term. For hard drugs, it is twenty years for personal possession and a life sentence if they think the stuff is intended for dealing. Bail is denied anyone busted on a drug charge. Before the revision, that was only the case for murder.

Following a contested presidential election in 2007, widespread ethnic violence left hundreds dead and thousands displaced. The riots pitted the Kikuyu, who have dominated the political system since independence in 1963, against the traditionally excluded Luo and Kalenjin peoples. They ended when the incumbent President Mwai Kibaki worked out a power-sharing deal with his Luo challenger Raila Odinga. But tensions persist. A Kikuyu extremist cult called the Mungiki carries out ritual beheadings and mutilations of their enemies. In Nairobi's slums, a Luo vigilante force with the unappetizing name of "Taliban" has emerged to fight them. One such district in Nairobi is such a war zone that it has won the name "Kosovo." In June 2007, when a suicide blast in the middle of a Nairobi street left one dead and dozens injured, authorities weren't sure if it was the Mungiki or Islamic extremists infiltrating from war-torn Somalia.

THE DOPE

Known variously as *kaya*, *iley*, *calley*, and *bhang*, cannabis is widely used in Kenya—despite its highly illegal status—and the UN Office on Drugs and Crimes notes that the country is becoming a major regional producer.

Street dealers abound in Nairobi and operate with surprising openness—and the dope is very cheap by Western standards. The strongest cannabis reportedly comes from the highlands around Mt. Kenya and Mt. Kilimanjaro. However, the stuff you get on the street may be adulterated—when it is called "special," that means it has been dipped in gasoline in a very misguided attempt to increase potency.

People wait with their belongings at a camp for internally displaced people at Tigoni police station west of Nairobi, Kenya. 2008 saw widespread violence between the Luo and Kikuyu peoples.

Dope Sheet

THE PRODUCT: The most potent varieties come from the Highlands, although this may be hard to find in Nairobi.

LOOK OUT FOR: Visit any one of the national parks for a look at Africa's game; trekking to the peak of Mount Kilimanjaro; Storymoja Hay Festival for folk tales and bands from many parts of East Africa.

FIRING SQUADS IN INDONESIA

Indonesia has some of the strictest drug laws on earth. The most celebrated case is that of Schapelle Corby, a young Australian woman serving a 20-year sentence for the importation of over 9 pounds (about 4 kilograms) of cannabis into Bali.

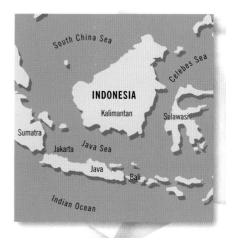

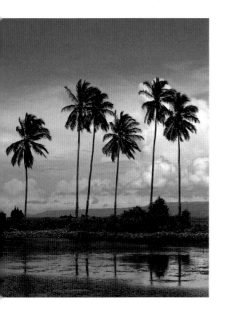

Palm trees and a blue lagoon; it's no surprise that Bali and many of its neighboring islands have become a popular destination for tourists from around the world.

She was convicted in May 2005 and by 2008 she had exhausted all of her possible appeals. If she serves the whole sentence, she will be 48 when she is released (although sentences are sometimes reduced on major national holidays). She refuses to plead for clemency because this would mean admitting guilt. From day one, she has maintained her innocence, saying the dope was planted on her. She says on her support website: "When I flew to Bali on 8 October 2004, I imagined my biggest problem was going to be deciding which sarong to wear with which bikini." But it could have been worse, believe it or not. Indonesian prosecutors initially vowed to send her to the firing squad.

THE HIGHS

Despite grim tales such as Corby's, there are many reasons to visit the country. The Indonesian archipelago is made up of more than 17,500 islands, stretching nearly 3,500 miles (5,500 kilometers) between the Pacific and Indian Oceans, right on the Equator. Most of the islands are uninhabited. Over half the nation's people live in the island of Java, where the capital Jakarta is. At Demak, the Grand Mosque—uniquely blending Hindu and Islamic architecture— dates to the first Muslim kingdom established on the island in 1511. Ancient temples from the earlier Hindu civilization can be seen at Borobudur. Traditional dance dramas or shadow-puppet shows are easy to find.

Just to the east lies Bali, a much smaller island, which contains the last surviving remnant of the archipelago's old Hindu culture—as well as a big tourist beach scene.

Some of the best surfing in the world is on the western side of the island. The town of Ubud in the island's center draws bohemian-type backpackers from around the globe. At the nearby Sacred Monkey Forest Sanctuary, you can watch macaques lounging around temples built specially for them. The Bali fire dance, an ancient Hindu tradition that has become something of a tourist spectacle, can be seen at the Uluwato temple.

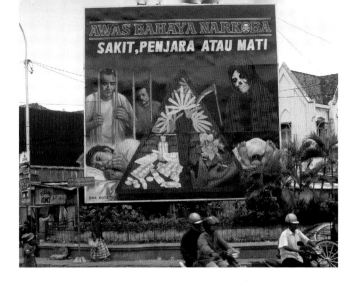

The next island to the east, Lombok, is a better-kept secret among surfers and scruffy backpackers, and is much more low-key and inexpensive. It is also less developed and has great views of the jungle coast from the interior mountains.

THE LOWS

Indonesian law imposes the death penalty for narcotics trafficking and up to twenty years for marijuana possession—even one to five years for personal quantities. The country just recently ended a four-year hiatus on the death penalty for drug offenses, which had been instated

pending clemency appeals and a constitutional review of the practice. Two Nigerians were executed by firing squad on June 16 2009—the International Day Against Drug Abuse and Illicit Trafficking—after being convicted of heroin smuggling.

Among those whose attorneys had demanded the constitutional review are three Australians sentenced to death for trying to smuggle heroin off Bali. Unfortunately, the Constitutional Court ruled that a constitutional amendment upholding the "right to life" did not

This antidrugs billboard in Yogyakarta, the main tourist destination in Java, reads "Sickness, Jail, or Death."

The 9th-century Buddhist temple compound at Borobudur is one of the greatest monuments in the world.

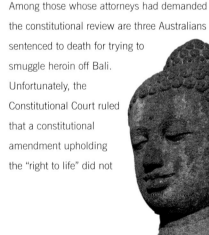

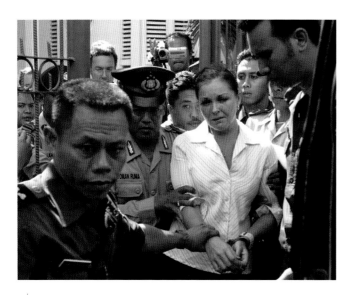

🌿 *Australian Schapelle Corby faces 20 years in prison after being found guilty of trying to smuggle 9 pounds (4 kilograms) of marijuana into Bali.*

🌿 *A man from Aceh holds up a marijuana leaf.*

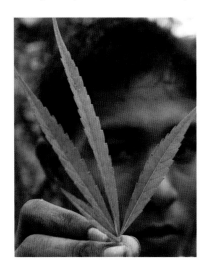

policy makes for a paranoid atmosphere. Further contributing to it are reports of police raiding nightclubs, blocking the exits, and conducting sweeps of the patrons. When police raided the Iguana disco in Medan, Sumatra, in 2005, many local youths jumped through the club's plate-glass windows. The club is on an upper floor of a department store, so there were several deaths and dozens injured.

As a tourist you'll encounter the usual problems with rip-offs and tourism parasites. One source calls the "neon-techno" scene at Bali's Kuta Beach a "great place to get set up and ripped off and sent on a bad deal."

apply to capital punishment. It should be pointed out that Indonesia executed only three in 2006, the year before the challenge was filed—compared with 53 in the USA that year, albeit not for drug trafficking. By way of comparison, China executed an estimated 1,000 that year; Iran executed 177; and Pakistan 82.

While there are 112 convicts on death row in Indonesia, it doesn't seem to be cutting down the local drug use. According to Health Ministry statistics, 18 million of the country's 238 million people are classified as "addicts." You can imagine that this

There have been a string of terrorist attacks over recent years. The October 2002 attack at Kuta left 200 dead. Twin bombings at Kuta and Jimbaran left another 23 dead in October 2005. In July 2009, nine were killed in a bomb attack on a business convention at Jakarta's Ritz-Carlton and Marriott hotels. A cell known as Jemaa Islamiyah is said to be behind the attacks. Several of its leaders are in prison or on trial, but the network is evidently alive.

There are simmering conflicts on all the major outer islands. Rebels demanding local rule are active in West Papua and have harassed the operations of the Freeport mining giant there. Aceh, at the northern tip of Sumatra, was the scene of a brutal war between the government and separatist guerillas. A peace deal was brokered after the 2004 tsunami devastated the region, but tensions persist. There has been some very nasty ethnic conflict between Muslims and Christians on Sulawesi. Kalimantan (Indonesian Borneo) has seen clashes between indigenous peoples and settlers from other islands.

THE DOPE

Indonesia is a major transshipment point for all things illicit, so there is cannabis and hashish from all over Asia there. However, dried brown stuff dominates the market. Much good local cannabis is grown in Aceh, and Indonesia is seeking US aid to instate a crop-substitution program there based on those that Washington uses against coca in Colombia and opium in Afghanistan. In an illustration of the absurdity of the

Dope Sheet

THE PRODUCT: Marijuana and hash from all over Asia pass through Indonesia; the best-quality ganja is grown in Aceh.

LOOK OUT FOR: Borobudur, Java, is one of the most spectacular religious complexes in the world; miles of sandy beaches; Bali for some excellent surfing; Sacred Monkey Forest Sanctuary; Uluwato temple for the Bali fire dance; head to Lombok for a more laid-back, low-key vibe.

prohibition regime, in 2007, Vice-President Yusuf Kalla publicly stated there was "no way" Indonesia would ever decriminalize—but in the same breath suggested that chefs who use the herb as a traditional curry seasoning should be exempt from the law! Evidently, he didn't get the word that you can get more stoned ingesting it than smoking it.

Bali's intricate terraces of rice paddies are spectacular, with many perched on the sides of steep hills.

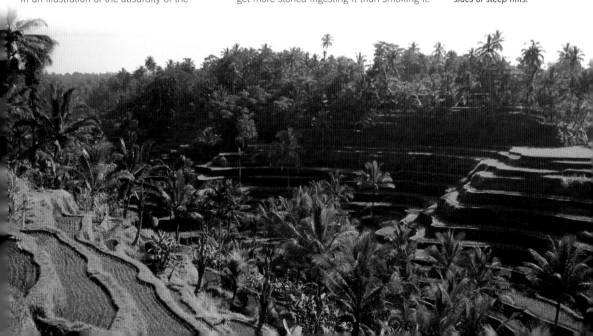

RESOURCES

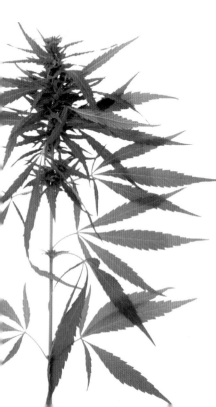

ORGANIZATIONS
HUMAN & CIVIL RIGHTS

NATIONAL ORGANIZATION FOR THE REFORM OF MARIJUANA LAWS (NORML)

1600 K Street, NW

Washington, DC 20006-2832

888-67-NORML (888-676-6765)

http://www.norml.org/

MARIJUANA POLICY PROJECT

236 Massachusetts Ave., NE

Washington, DC 20002

202-462-5747

http://www.mpp.org/

DRUG POLICY ACTION NETWORK

70 West 36th Street

New York, NY 10018

212-613-8020

http://www.dpa.convio.net/

STOP THE DRUG WAR

1623 Connecticut Ave., NW

Washington, DC 20009

202-293-8340

http://www.stopthedrugwar.org/

CRIMINAL JUSTICE POLICY FOUNDATION

8730 Georgia Avenue

Silver Spring, MD 20910

301-589-6020

http://www.cjpf.org/

STUDENTS FOR SENSIBLE DRUG POLICY

1623 Connecticut Ave, NW

Washington, DC 20009

202-293-4414

http://www.ssdp.org/

UK CANNABIS INTERNET ACTIVISTS (CIA)

The Greenhouse

Bethel Street

Norwich NR1 1NR, UK

http://www.ukcia.org/

AMNESTY INTERNATIONAL

1 Easton Street

London WC1X 0DW, UK

http://www.amnesty.org/

TRAVEL, ADVENTURE & FUN

CANNABIS CUP WINNERS

http://www.cannabiscupwinners.com/

BARCELONA SPANNABIS

http://www.spannabis.com/

VANSTERDAM GANJA GAMES

http://www.vansterdambowl.com/

GLASTONBURY FESTIVALS

http://www.glastonburyfestivals.co.uk/

REGGAE RISING, HUMBOLDT, CA

http://www.ReggaeRising.com/

REGGAE ON THE RIVER, HUMBOLDT, CA

http://www.mateel.org/

GREAT MIDWEST MARIJUANA HARVEST FESTIVAL

http://www.madisonhempfest.com/

SEATTLE HEMPFEST

http://www.hempfest.org/

TORONTO FREEDOM FESTIVAL

http://www.torontofreedomfestival.com/

NIMBIN MARDIGRASS

http://www.NimbinMardiGrass.com/

RAINBOW FAMILY OF LIVING LIGHT

http://www.welcomehome.org/

RAINBOW PRESS CREW

http://www.rpcnews.us/

BETHEL WOODS CENTER FOR THE ARTS

http://www.bethelwoodscenter.org/

THE PACIFIC COAST OF MEXICO

http://www.tomzap.com/

PUBLICATIONS

WEBSITES

GLOBAL GANJA REPORT

http://www.globalganjareport.com/

WORLD WAR 4 REPORT

http://www.ww4report.com/

NARCO NEWS

http://www.narconews.com/

UPSIDE DOWN WORLD

http://www.upsidedownworld.org/

DRUGWAR.COM

http://www.drugwar.com/

HIGH TIMES

http://www.hightimes.com/

BOOKS

THE CANNABIS COMPANION

Steve Wishnia

(Running Press, 2004)

**ORGIES OF THE HEMP EATERS:
CUISINE, SLANG, LITERATURE
& RITUAL OF CANNABIS CULTURE**

Hakim Bey & Abel Zug, editors

(Autonomedi, 2004)

**MARIHUANA: THE FIRST
TWELVE THOUSAND YEARS**

Ernest L. Abel

(Plenum Press, 1980)

MARIHUANA RECONSIDERED

Lester Grinspoon, MD

(Quick American Archives, 1994)

**PEOPLE OF THE RAINBOW:
A NOMADIC UTOPIA**

Michael I. Niman

(University of Tennessee Press, 1997)

**RAINBOW NATION WITHOUT BORDERS:
TOWARD AN ECOTOPIAN MILLENNIUM**

Alberto Ruz Buenfil

(Bear & Co., 1991)

THE PEOPLE'S GUIDE TO MEXICO

Carl Franz & Lorena Havens

(Avalon Travel Publishing, 2006)

**HOMAGE TO CHIAPAS: THE NEW
INDIGENOUS STRUGGLES IN MEXICO**

Bill Weinberg

(Verso Books, 2000)

**HOW DE BODY? ONE MAN'S TERRIFYING
JOURNEY THROUGH AN AFRICAN WAR**

Teun Voeten

(Thomas Dunne Publishing, 2002)

A TRAVELLER'S HISTORY OF INDIA

Sinharaja Tammita-Delgoda

(Interlink Books, 2003)

**AFGHANISTAN (ESSENTIAL FIELD GUIDES
TO HUMANITARIAN AND CONFLICT ZONES)**

Edward Girardet & Jonathan Walter

(International Centre for Humanitarian
Reporting, 1998)

BARCELONA

Robert Hughes

(Alfred A. Knopf, 1992)

INDEX

ACKNOWLEDGMENTS

First and foremost, I'd like to thank my old *High Times* buds who are still burning the torch of freedom (as well as other things): Peter Gorman, John Veit, Steve Wishnia, Gabe Kirchheimer, Dean Latimer, Preston Peet, Steve Bloom, Chesley Hicks, and Sarah Ferguson. Next, my army of tireless interns: Lucille Flood, Iulia Anghelescu, Brooklyn Yimer, Stanley Yeung, and Anthony Portillo. Next, my general all-purpose support crew: Joe Wetmore and Karen Edelstein of Autumn Leaves Used Books in Ithaca, NY; Jim Fleming at Autonomedia; Jason Goodrow, Robbie Liben, Petros Korakis, and David Bloom. And, finally, my sources: Hakim Bey, Zero Boy, DJ Gringo Loco, Steve Ben Israel, Darryl Cherney, Maria Anguera de Sojo, Ben Masel, Travis Wendel, Derek Williams of UK Cannabis Internet Activists (UKCIA), Alan St Pierre of the National Organization for the Reform of Marijuana Laws (NORML), and Eric Sterling of the Criminal Justice Policy Foundation.

CREDITS

Mary Jane by Rick James was first released by Gordy (Motown) in 1978. The Ivy Press would like to thank all of the individuals and organizations who contributed images to this project, without whom this book wouldn't have been possible:

Alamy/Bikem Ekberzade: 11; David Hoffman: 64b; Phil Rees: 64t; Cristian Baitg Reportage: 70, 71; Jeffrey Blackler: 86b; Friedrich Stark: 88; JTB Photo Communications, Inc: 90b; BrazilPhotos.com: 98; Jon Arnold Images Ltd: 115. T.J. Bissonnette: 101b. Bridgeman Art Library/Bibliotheque Nationale, Paris, France/Archives Charmet: 67t. Donna B. Cooper: 100, 101t. Corbis/Roger Ressmeyer: 25t; Jorge Uzon: 35; Xavier Bertral/epa: 51b; Marcel Antonisse/epa: 60b; Allen Ginsberg: 67b; Ed Kashi: 72, 74t; Reinhard Eisele: 89b; Howard Davies: 90t; Daniel Lainé: 91; Michele Falzone/JAI: 93b; Karen Huntt: 94 Michele Falzone/JAI: 95; Pascale Mariani/Romeo Langlois: 105t, 105b; Danny Lehman: 108; Mario Guzman/epa: 110t; John Brecher: 110b; Pascal Manoukian/Sygma: 112; Reuters: 113; Jon Hrusa/epa: 119. Dominic Cramer/Toronto Hemp Company: 33t. Jonathan Cronin: 45b. Fotolia/Renáta Sedmáková: 10; Mat Hayward: 17b; EvilGirl: 33b; Claus Mikosch: 57t; Cepesh: 62; Julien Sarrazin: 69t; Geoffrey Métais: 73; Wolszczak: 77; Diorgi: 78t; Impala: 80; Yeti: 81; Alexander Mandl: 82b, 83; thawizard: 84; Celso Pupo: 97t; Jerome Dancette: 97b; Delli-Pizzi: 114; Javarman: 118. Scott Gacek: 53. Alexander Gaylon: 39b. Getty Images: 14, 15l, 15r; Owen Franken: 60t; AFP: 69b; 93t; AFP: 99; De Agostini: 104; 106; AFP: 107; 109t; Kyle George: 111; AFP: 116, 117; 122t; AFP: 122b. Mark Graham: 47. Grandmasterka: 37. Tim Grant: 76. Justin Holzworth: 16. Hypersapiens: 34. iStockphoto/Gregory Olsen: 17t; FotoVoyager: 20; Constantgardener: 24; David Freund: 40; VikaValter: 48; Matthew Dixon: 49; John Woodcock: 57b; Devy Masselink: 58b; Justin Horrocks: 59b; Sean Randall: 68; David Garry: 74b; Sandeep Subba: 82t; Brytta: 85; Jakob Leitner: 86t; Cathleen Abers-Kimball: 89t; Zazen Photography: 121b; Klaus Hollitzer: 123. Jeremiah Leif Johnson: 38, 39t, 124. Jupiter Images: 2, 29b, 32, 36, 52b, 58c, 59t, 87, 109b. Jean-Michel Just: 65. Gabe Kirchheimer: 28, 30t, 30b, 31. Luna Creative: 21. MassCann/NORML: 52t. Jon Mulhern: 22; Kate Newton - kate.newton@gmail.com: 41t, 41b, 42t, 42b, 43, 56. Javier Perez Vera: 50b, 51t. Mickie Quick: 121t. Jonny Reimer: 78b. Tony Rocha - http://www.flickr.com/photos/aerocha: 25b, 26t, 26b, 27. Tristan Savatier: 44, 45t, 46T. Scuddr: 63. Markane Sipraseuth: 18, 19. Rafa Siquier: 61. Christopher Soghoain: 79. Spannabis: 50, 125. Topfoto/The Granger Collection: 10t; Roger-Viollet: 66. Arturo Torres: 75. Swiatoslaw Woitkowiak: 46b. Antonia Zabala: 92.